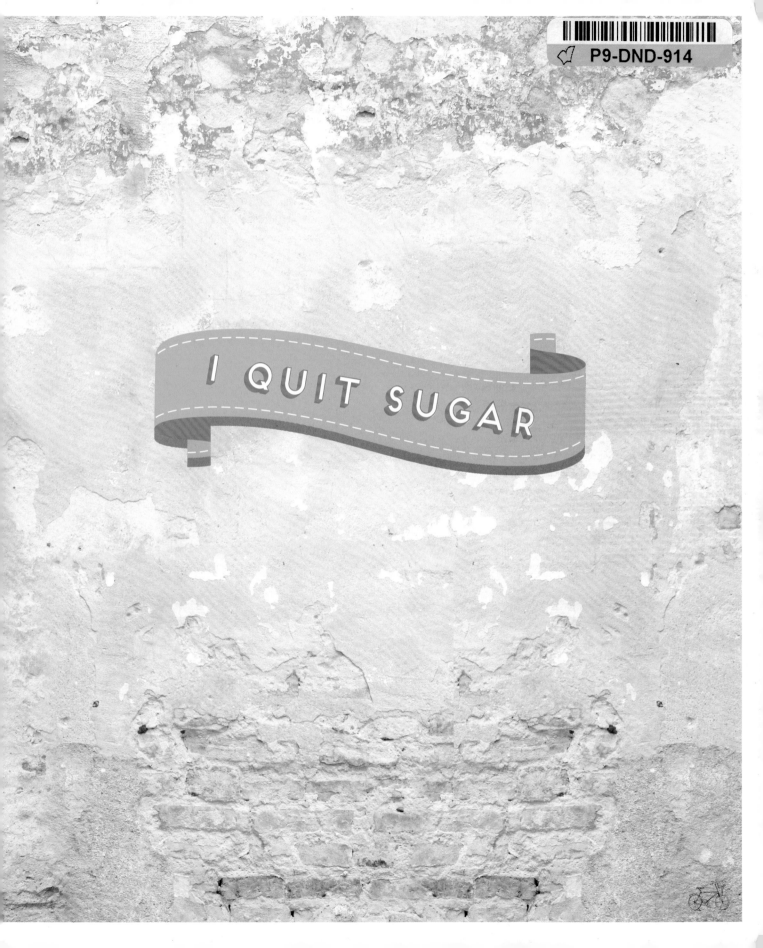

I QUIT SUGAR

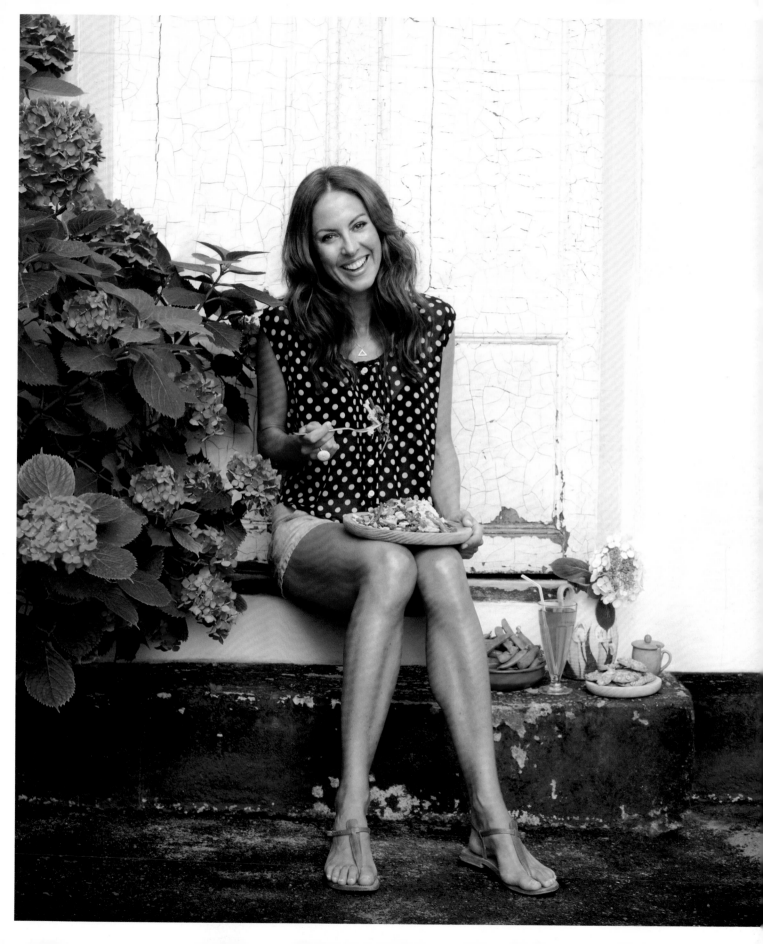

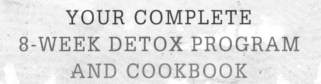

I QUIT SUGAR

YOUR COMPLETE
8-WEEK DETOX PROGRAM
AND COOKBOOK

SARAH WILSON

CLARKSON POTTER/PUBLISHERS
NEW YORK

A LITTLE DEDICATION

I wrote this for everyone who's ever struggled with their eating
and their health. And then given themselves a stinkin' hard time
for not finding a way to get on top of things.
And I wish to say to you all:

YOU'RE NOT ALONE.

WE'RE ALL IN THIS TOGETHER.

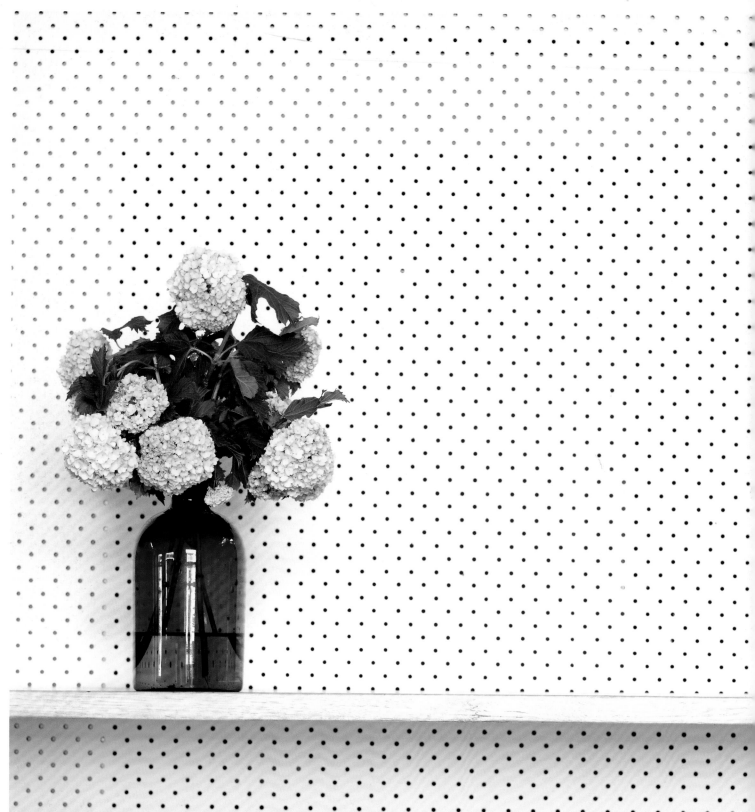

CONTENTS

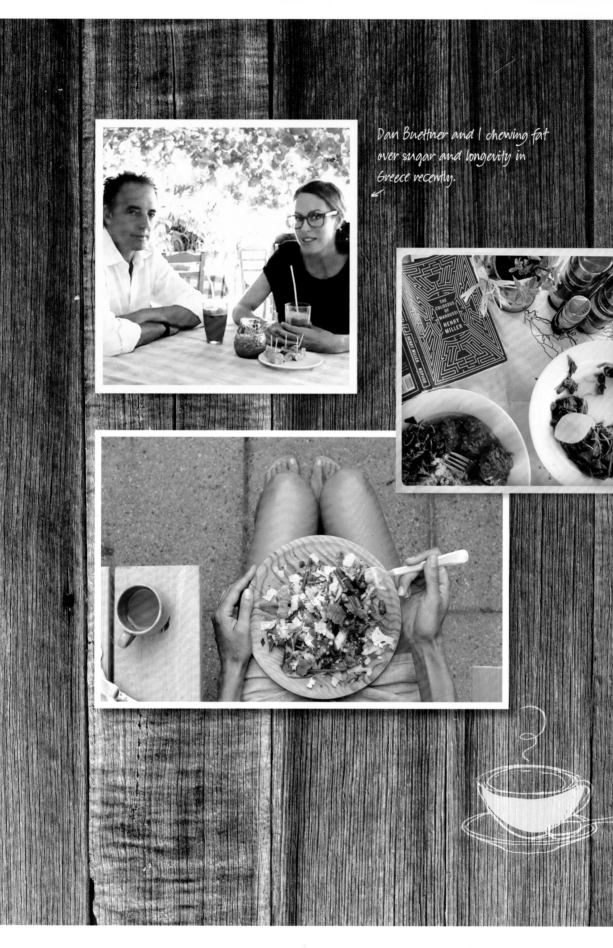

Dan Buettner and I chewing fat over sugar and longevity in Greece recently.

by Dan Buettner

**National Geographic Fellow and *New York Times*
best-selling author of *The Blue Zones: Lessons for
Living Longer from the People Who've Lived the Longest***

What should you eat? I just Googled "diet" and
was presented with 656 million results. WebMD
scientifically reviews 94 diets—everything from the
"Atkins Diet" to the "Zone Diet"; from the "Gene Smart
Diet" to the "Cookie Diet." Here's the bottom line:
None of them work! Sure, any one of them will help
you lose weight for a few weeks or a few months. But
we humans are hardwired for variety and pretty soon,
no matter how seemingly fantabulous a new diet may
seem, we're going to get bored with it and stray. I defy
anyone to tell me about a diet that has worked for more
than two years.

I've spent over a decade studying what centenarians
eat to be 100 and I can tell you a few things for sure.
First is that evolution provides important cues for
helping us decide what to eat. Think about what
your grandparents ate, the quantity, the level of
processing, the freshness, and you can get a pretty
good idea of what humans have been eating for the
past few centuries. Second, we all need to experiment
and find out what works for our lifestyle and our
particular body chemistry. I believe that vegetables
are good for you, but if I eat eggplant—and I don't
know why eggplant—the roof of my mouth swells like
a sea anemone. Third, if we eat what we like, we're
going to probably eat it for long enough to make a real
difference in our health—for better or for worse.

Which is why I like Sarah Wilson's approach to
eating, and particularly this book. Sarah is a food

explorer of the highest order. She began her deep dive
into the science of eating not because she wanted
to sell books, but because she had an intrinsically
personal and authentic motive: she needed to heal
herself. She then proceeded with journalistic rigor
and Machiavellian resolve to get to primary sources of
dietary information. She's personally interviewed the
top scientists and/or has metabolized their research to
produce a powerful understanding of how food impacts
our wellness (I call her a walking Googlet of Dietary
Information). Then she traveled the world in search of
recipes that match her best practices. Couple this with
her epicurean sensibilities and the fact that she started
cooking at an age when most kids are learning to walk,
you have the perfect credentials to write a cookbook.
My advice: Take a Sarah Wilsonesque expedition of your
own through the pages of this book. Try most of these
recipes, turn your favorites into weekly habits, and
watch wellness ensue!

P.S. Dan and I met after I wrote about
his Blue Zone theories a few years ago.
We started a robust electronic dialogue
over our common interests—mountain
biking, eating and exploring. I love that
he digs my book! Sarah

Sharing a sugar-free treat!

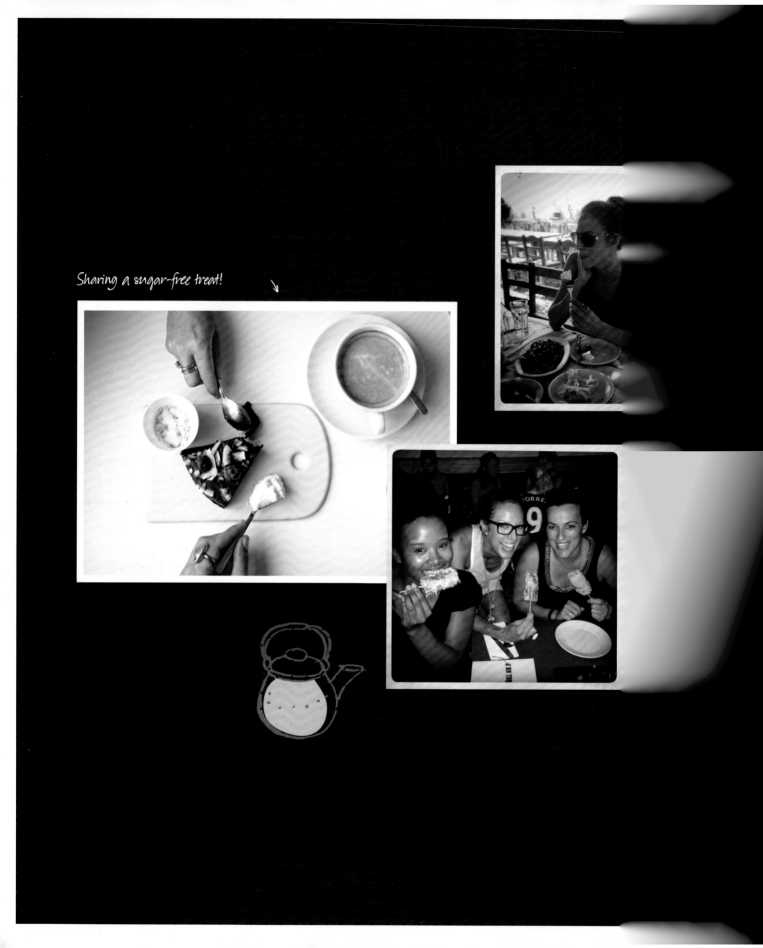

INTRODUCTION

THREE YEARS AGO
I DECIDED TO QUIT SUGAR.
I'd played with the idea many
times before, but had never
quite gone the full distance.
Then I decided to get serious.

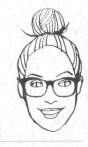

What started out as just a New Year experiment became something more. Giving up sugar was easier than I thought, and I felt better than ever, so I just kept going and going.

I interviewed dozens of experts around the world and did my own research as a qualified health coach. I experimented, using myself as a guinea pig, and eventually assembled a stack of scientifically tested techniques that really worked. Then I got serious and committed. I chose.

THESE THINGS ARE ALWAYS A MATTER OF CHOOSING.

AND COMMITTING.

We have a deep-rooted resistance to quitting sugar. We grow up with an emotional and physical attachment to it. Just the idea of not being able to turn to it when we're feeling happy or want to celebrate, or when we're feeling low or tired, terrifies us.

If not a sweet treat, then what? Well, I'll tell you what:

A MIND AND BODY THAT'S CLEAN AND CLEAR.

But I soon learned that when you quit sugar, you can feel very much on your own. Our modern food system is set up around sugar, and seductively so. A granola bar can contain more sugar than a block of chocolate; everyday barbeque sauce, more than chocolate topping. You try to do the right thing only to find low-fat yogurt contains more sugar than ice cream. You feed your kids "whole grain" cereal in the morning with some juice and pack their lunchbox with "healthy" snacks, like raisins or fruit. By lunch, they've eaten their way through a Milky Way-bar-and-cola-can-worth of sugar.

And don't try taking refuge in a health food shop—they're little dens of fructose-dressed-up-as-healthy-foodstuffs. Some of the highest fructose snacks I've encountered were found in health food shops, usually festooned with "low fat," "gluten-free," "100% natural" and even "no added sugar" labels. What hope do we have?

It also doesn't help that the nutritional bodies we rely on to advise us as to what to put in our mouths are in many cases funded by—you guessed it—the sugar industry.

JUST ABOUT EVERYTHING WE EAT IS LACED WITH SUGAR.

I found breakfast became a minefield and trying to grab a healthy, sugar-free snack on the run was virtually impossible. I had to get clever and creative. So I spent the next twelve months inventing new fructose-free snacks and meals, both sweet and sweet-diverting.

THIS BOOK WILL SHOW YOU HOW TO TAKE SUGAR OUT OF YOUR DIET AND GET WELL.

▶ It's a step-by-step eight-week program, full of tips, tricks and techniques that will help you eliminate the white stuff for good.

PLUS IT'S A RECIPE BOOK

▶ It's a compendium of all the things that I personally ate and treated myself to while giving up sugar, and ever since. The recipes are a combination of my "inventions," plus a few contributions from some of my lovely health-focused friends.

For me, eating sugar-free has become incredibly easy, efficient, economical, sustainable and . . . right.

For the first time in decades, I am eating exactly what I want. That's what going sugar-free does—it recalibrates your appetite. I don't think about restricting my intake. Ever. And eating has become even more joyous and deeply, wholly satiating.

I'm no white-coated expert. But I did succeed in ridding my life of sugar and I did experience first-hand what worked and what didn't. Now I want to share what I found and help as many people as I can make the leap to healthy, sugar-free living.

I wish you luck and a whole lot of wellness.

Sarah XX

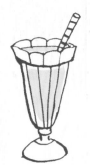

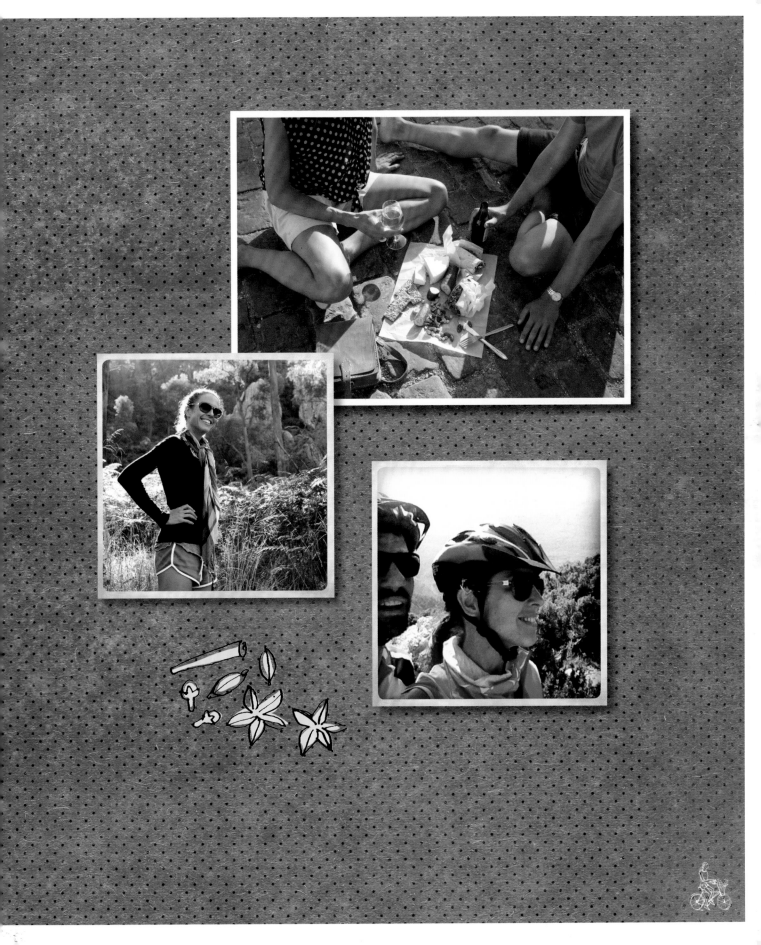

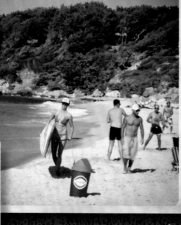

I eat to surf. And hike . . . ↑

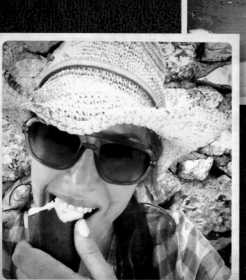

↑ My very un-fancy hiking snack of choice: the cucumber.

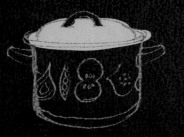

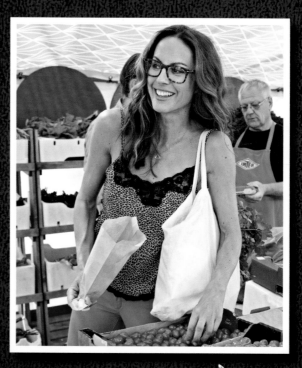

I shop every few days, as I need things. ↑
I cook with what I have in the fridge.

JUST A FEW THINGS ABOUT THE RECIPES

The recipes in this book are not fancy. They're simple and everyday.

Less is more. I try to use as few ingredients as possible. You'll notice that I use the same staples over and over throughout the book. This way you get to experiment with each ingredient, using it in a number of different ways, plus it means you're not buying an entire jar of something for one dish, never to be used again. This means less waste—which is fundamental these days, right?

I don't like to cook precisely. The recipes reflect this and, as a result, are really rather foolproof. See them as an invitation to play a little and experiment.

I focus on stumbling blocks. When you give up sugar, the hardest foods to accommodate are breakfasts, quick-and-easy snacks, desserts and feeding your kids—which is why I've focused squarely on these. I've also provided some great detox meals that will help with the transition period to sugar-free eating.

Most of the recipes are completely fructose-free and are perfect for the eight-week quit-sugar program.

Some contain sugar alternatives or low-fructose fruits and are best for eating after the two-month quitting period.

The recipes are mostly gluten- and grain-free because I think starches from grains can feed the sugar addiction and are best minimized if you have issues with sugar.

The recipes are mostly suitable for those with fructose malabsorption, but some people with that condition can't eat coconut products. It's worth speaking with a nutritionist or doctor about this if you're concerned.

This is not strictly a Paleo cookbook, mostly because I don't subscribe to dietary labels. The principle of the Paleolithic diet is that we should eat as close to the way our hunter-gather ancestors did 10,000 years ago—lots of meat, fat, nuts, vegetables, and some fruit, and no grains or sugar. Most of the recipes in this book are Paleo-suitable, but with some great vegetarian and vegan options provided.

When a recipe calls for dairy, meat or eggs, please try to use free-range, pasture- or grass-fed, organic options. Not so flush with cash? Try cheaper, less fashionable cuts of meat, and don't trim the fat, bones and cartilage. Use them instead to make a stock (see page 60).

These recipes are a reflection of how I cook. I like to mix a bit of this and that. I eat whole (never low-fat), nutrient-dense food where possible.

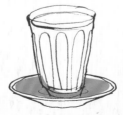

I WAS A SUGAR ADDICT.
I DIDN'T LOOK LIKE ONE.
I didn't drink Coke or put sugar in my coffee. I've never eaten a Krispy Kreme donut, and ice cream bores me.

BUT HERE'S THE THING: I WAS A COVERT ADDICT.

I hid behind the so-called "healthy sugars" like honey, dark chocolate and fruit. Which made things harder in some ways because first I had to face my denial.

Growing up on a simple, self-sufficient property, my family ate very naturally. My attachment started when, as a teenager, I moved into town from the country. A cocktail of girl hormones, newfound access to malls and convenience stores, as well as a-kid-in-candy-store delight with foods I'd previously been denied meant I went sugar crazy.

I remember not being able to function at university if I didn't have a cinnamon bun at 10 a.m. I loved the icing and convinced myself the dried currants made it healthy.

Over time this wasn't enough. I'd then eat an apple pie after lunch. And some chocolate. Soon, I was riding a horrible roller coaster of sugar highs and lows. I was bingeing. Then, feeling guilty, I would starve myself the rest of the day.

I got sick as a result of this reactionary eating—very sick. I developed mood disorders and sleep problems, and finally I developed adrenal issues and my first autoimmune disease—Graves, or overactive thyroid. Ever since, I've had stomach problems linked to poor digestive balance and have developed further autoimmune issues, most recently Hashimoto's.

Over time I swapped my processed sugary carbs for "healthy" sugary treats. And, yeah, I ate less sugar overall. But all the symptoms still continued. I didn't put it down to sugar completely. But I knew it was a major player.

For the past eleven years I've eaten very well. But up until three years ago I was still eating too much sugar every day. After every meal. I was still addicted.

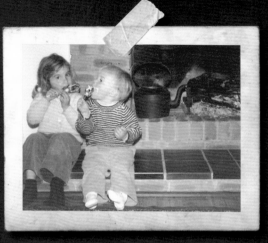

As a kid I liked to supervise the cooking . . .
and lick the beaters with my brother Ben.

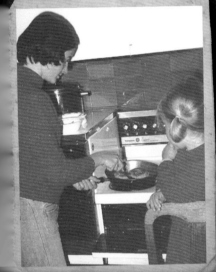

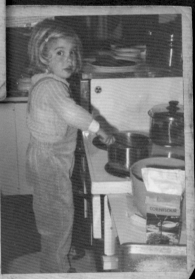

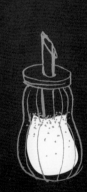

SO HOW ADDICTED WAS I?

A conservative day would see me consume about **25+** teaspoons of sugar

HERE'S A SNAPSHOT:

I was eating three pieces of fruit a day, a handful of dried fruit, a teaspoon or two of honey in my tea, a small (1.2 oz.) bar of dark chocolate after lunch and, after dinner, honey drizzled on yogurt, or dessert (if I was out).

A conservative day would see me consume about 25-plus teaspoons of sugar, just in that rundown of snacks above. That's not counting the hidden sugar in things like tomato sauce and commercial breads.

I told myself I ate "good" sugar and convinced myself I didn't have a problem.

BUT SUGAR IS SUGAR.

Sure, the other ingredients mixed in with the sugar in, say, a granola bar or a piece of fruit were good for me. But the chemical composition of sugar—whether it's in a mango or a chocolate bar—remains the same. And it is highly addictive.

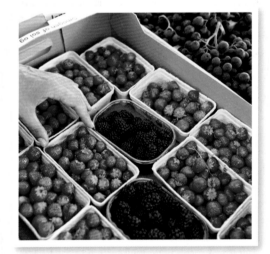

IT WAS TIME TO FACE THE FACTS.

FACT 1: I WAS EATING WAY MORE SUGAR THAN WE'RE DESIGNED TO EAT.

Even though I was eating much less sugar than the average person, and many would say my diet looked very healthy, I was still consuming too much sugar.

Q: How much sugar are we meant to eat, again?

As little as possible is the simple answer. The longer answer is more convoluted and there are many diverging opinions on intake and what constitutes sugar and, indeed, added sugar. Regardless, the take-home is this: *Around the world, recommendations are increasingly being revised down and down . . . which suggests something, right?* The American Heart Association recommends no more than 6 teaspoons (24 grams) a day for women, 9 teaspoons (36 grams) for men and 3 teaspoons (12 grams) for kids.

Where does this leave us? As a general rule, I simply try to keep my sugar intake as low as possible. If pressed for a limit? I work toward what many argue is the amount we ate back when our metabolisms were forming 10,000 years ago, derived from a few pieces of fruit and starches. It's an imprecise but useful target: *6–9 teaspoons of added sugar a day is my recommended limit.*

FACT 2: I WAS ADDICTED.

And in a most undignified way. If someone put a cheesecake in front of me or a family-sized block of chocolate, and I was having a weak moment, I'd damn well eat the whole thing. Once I got a taste, I couldn't control myself.

FACT 3: AUTOIMMUNE DISEASE (*OR ADRENAL ISSUES OR AN EXCITABLE PERSONALITY*) + SUGAR = BAD.

I suspect my autoimmune disease is, to an extent, linked to my lifelong sugar habit. And it is certainly made worse by sugar. Anyone with a compromised system simply cannot afford to have their stress hormones (adrenaline and cortisol), their neurotransmitter levels (dopamine), or their insulin levels tipped off balance by sugar. It's a hard, cold, but oddly motivating fact!

FACT 4: I WANTED TO LOSE WEIGHT.

I'd put on weight (26 lb.) from my thyroid disease a few years back and hadn't been able to drop it. It wasn't a core issue for me but it played on my mind. I was eager to see if cutting sugar would help.

FACT 5: I'D HAD ENOUGH.

I was done with riding the roller coaster of sugar highs and lows and my obsession with my next fix. And I figured it was time to at least try eliminating sugar. Just to see what happened.

To begin with, I committed to "just trying it out." But after two weeks I felt so much clearer and cleaner, I kept going. I wasn't draconian about it. I just remained curious . . .

This is a principle I apply to many aspects of my life. Like exercise. I commit to exercising 20 minutes every day (it's the "every day" bit that counts). I don't balk at the idea of 20 minutes, so I do it without fuss. Plus, once I set out for a jog or a swim for 20 minutes, I get engaged and invariably go for a bit longer. I apply the same psychology to quitting sugar. It works!

NOTE

WE ARE DESIGNED TO EAT 6–9 TEASPOONS OF SUGAR A DAY.

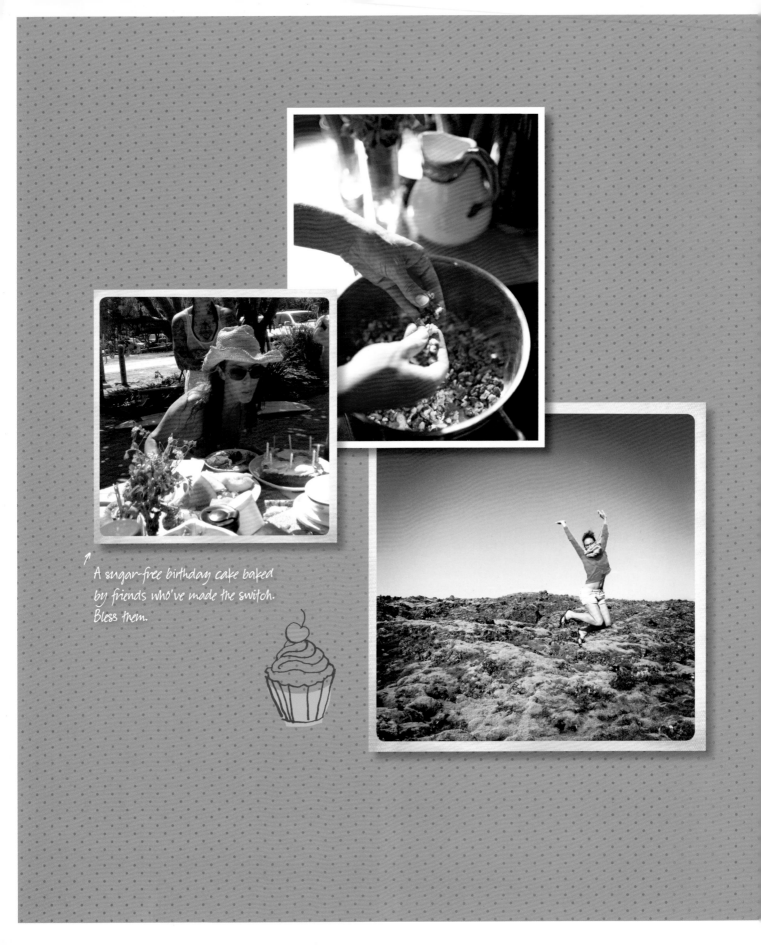

A sugar-free birthday cake baked
by friends who've made the switch.
Bless them.

I'LL BE UP-FRONT.
There are a few harsh-ish realities to bear in mind before you set out:

▶ **Quitting, I found, took about two months.** Studies say it takes between 21 and 66 days to change a habit from a *psychological* perspective. My experience and research found it took most people the same amount of time to overcome the physical habit of eating sugar, too. Sugar is a gnarly habit; I advise pacing yourself. Do it properly over eight weeks.

▶ **When you first quit sugar, you must quit ALL of it.** Including fruit, fruit juice, agave and honey. Some nutritionists advise just cutting out the added sugar. But a lot of the sugar experts agree: it's best to get rid of all of it at first, so you can break the addiction and then recalibrate.

▶ **At the end of the eight-week program,** some fruit and safe table sugar alternatives can be reintroduced.

▶ **There is a detox period where you will feel like crap.** This lasted only a week or two for me. For some it can last six weeks. After that, it's a non-issue. I promise.

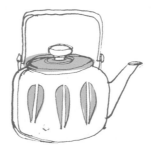

FIRST CONSIDER THIS:

▶ We're eating more low-fat food than ever before.

▶ We're joining more gyms.

▶ Yet we're putting on more weight.

THEN CONSIDER THIS:

▶ Today we eat more than 2 pounds of sugar a week. Just 150 years ago we ate next to none.

▶ Low-fat food often contains more sugar than the wholefood version. (Sugar is added to make a food taste more like the original.)

▶ The low-fat industry is big business.

A PICTURE FORMS, RIGHT?

There is a lot of resistance to eliminating sugar. The sugar and corn industries in many countries are propped up by government tariffs. And government nutrition bodies around the world are too often funded by the sugar industry. I don't want to spell things out with outrage and finger-pointing. But I will highlight that quitting sugar is something that's not about to be encouraged by a big worldwide health initiative any time soon.

We have to make the change ourselves, consciously.

SHOULD YOU BE QUITTING?

▶ Do you get an energy slump in the afternoon?

▶ Do you need something sweet after meals?

▶ Does your stomach get bloated after eating?

▶ Are you unable to eat just one piece of cake and walk away?

▶ Are you pudgy around the middle, perhaps even slim everywhere else?

▶ Do you often feel unclear? That you're not always sharp and on-form?

I ticked "yes" to most of the above and had a sneaking suspicion that sugar might be the thing making me feel baseline-crappy. If you do too, then have a go and see if quitting works. It has for tens of thousands of people who have completed my eight-week program already. (Check out the testimonials on the inside covers of this book.)

We'll be following a few *I Quit Sugar* mantras throughout the program. This is the first.

IQS MANTRA 1

BE GENTLE AND KIND

As you do this program, please go gently and don't punish yourself.

We don't respond well to "restrictive thinking." You're doing this not because you have to, but because it might make you feel better. Be alive to this as often as you can through this process. Gentle and kind . . .

MY FINAL TIPS ON QUITTING

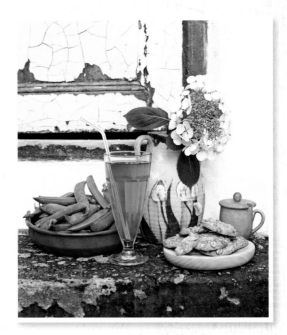

Take a "let's just see" approach and it will make the process less onerous.

Get an IQS buddy to do it with you. It does make it easier. Even just to have someone to cook new foods with.

Read and learn as much information on the science of sugar absorption and sugar politics as you can. It will help remind you why you're doing it, and keep you motivated. (See page 21 for ideas.)

Change doesn't happen with an about-face. It happens by building up habits in our minds. Slowly, we form new neural pathways in our brains until we're doing things differently, effortlessly. So every day that we flex our "I'm not eating sugar" muscle, the stronger we get. I found it helped to view this process as a strengthening exercise.

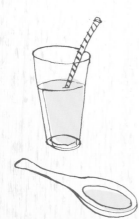

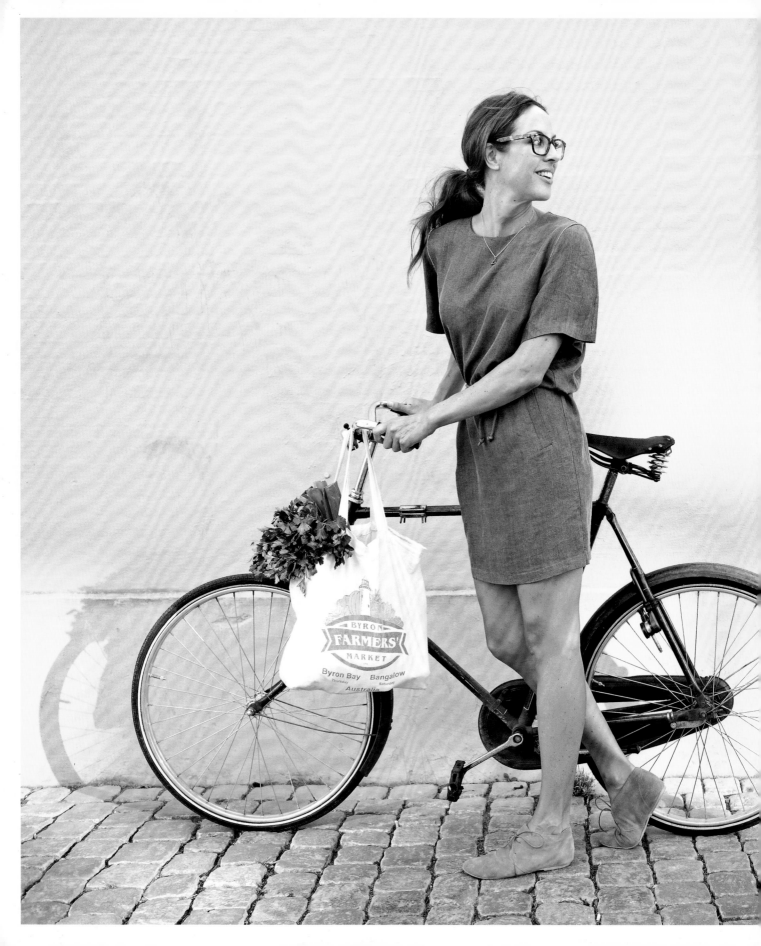

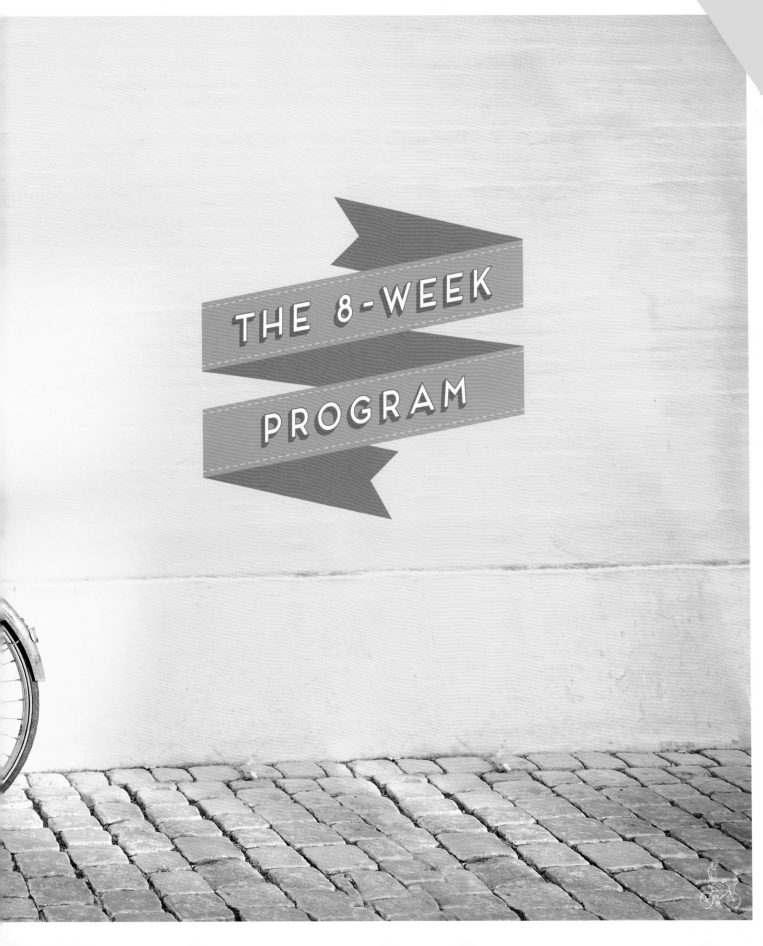

START TO CUT BACK

SOME EXPERTS ADVISE GOING COLD TURKEY FROM THE OUTSET.
Me, not so much.

This first week is about a few easy, simple changes that aren't too detailed or complicated. We're not going to cut out all sugar straightaway—I think it's worth having a little warm-up. My theory is that humans respond badly to outright bans. Tell me not to touch the "wet paint" and all I want to do is touch the wet paint. If we're told to stop eating a certain food, we'll crave it all the more and it's all we can think about.

THE LESS SUGAR IN YOUR SYSTEM BEFORE YOU ENTER WEEK 2, THE EASIER IT WILL BE.

Your digestive system will be in a better place to deal with the adjustment and the cravings will be milder. Stick to this experimental "I'm just playing with the idea" phase for one or two weeks. But not too long. You don't want to get bored with the experiment.

DO THIS

PARE BACK ON SUGAR.

And while you're at it, pare back on the refined carbohydrates (donuts, bready and white floury things, etc.). Start to become more food-conscious and make a few simple swaps:

▶ Toast with a few avocado slices, olive oil drizzled on top, and red pepper flakes, if you like, instead of toast with jam.

▶ Eggs on toast instead of granola and low-fat yogurt.

▶ Herbal tea or soda water instead of juice and soft drinks.

▶ Popcorn at the movies instead of a bag of candy.

▶ Cheese instead of dessert after dinner.

▶ If you drink sugar in your tea and coffee, halve the amount and add in extra milk (which tastes sweet, but contains no fructose). Or, only as an interim measure, use artificial sweetener instead. (I explain later why fake sugars are not a good idea. For now, to get you off sugar, we can live with a week or two of it, for adjustment purposes.)

▶ If you're addicted to soft drinks, swap to the diet versions—again, only as an interim measure. That is, for a week or two.

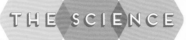
A few factoids to get started.

To be clear, it's fructose that's the enemy, not sugar, per se.

WHEN I TALK ABOUT QUITTING SUGAR, I'M TALKING ABOUT QUITTING FRUCTOSE.

And here's why it's bad!

1 Fructose makes us eat more.

Every molecule we put in our mouths has corresponding appetite hormones. And when we've eaten enough of said molecule, these hormones tell our brains, "We're full now; stop eating." Our bodies are good that way; we're designed to eat only as much as we need.

EVERY MOLECULE, THAT IS, EXCEPT FRUCTOSE.

This is because back when we were cave people, sugar was both highly valuable (as instant energy for chasing wildebeests) and extremely rare (a berry here and there). Thus we evolved with no fructose "full switch." This was so that when we did stumble on a berry bush, we could gorge ourselves stupid (and store it as instant fat).

All very well back when sugar was rare and we had to work hard to get it. But now it's ludicrously abundant and we barely have to extend an arm to get at it. Having no "off switch" is a massive liability!

2 Fructose converts directly to fat.

After eating fructose, most of the metabolic burden for metabolizing it rests on your liver. This is not the case with glucose, of which your liver breaks down only 20%. Nearly every cell in your body utilizes glucose, so it's normally "burned up" immediately after consumption. The way fructose is converted in our bodies means it's not used straightaway as energy, but converted directly to fat. When we drink fructose (in soft drinks and juices), this process is even more direct and faster.

3 Fructose makes us sick.

More and more research is being done on the effects of fructose on our bodies. A number of studies have found that fructose:

- inhibits our immune system, making it harder to fight off viruses and infections.
- upsets the mineral balance in our bodies, causing deficiencies as well as interfering with mineral absorption.
- messes with fertility.
- speeds up the aging process.
- has been connected with the development of cancers of the breast, ovaries, prostate, rectum, pancreas, lung, gallbladder and stomach.
- is linked to dementia.
- causes an acidic digestive tract, indigestion and malabsorption.
- can cause a rapid rise in adrenaline, as well as hyperactivity, anxiety and a loss of concentration.

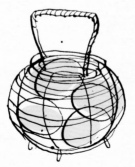

WEEK 1

SUGAR = POISON?

The research is growing to show sugar is indeed poisoning us. Studies are proving sugar to be the biggest cause of fatty liver, which leads to insulin resistance. This then causes metabolic syndrome, which is now being seen as the biggest precursor to heart disease, diabetes and cancer.

Sugar isn't just a bunch of naughty, empty calories. Some leading scientists are saying it's responsible for 35 million annual deaths worldwide.

GARY TAUBES, AUTHOR OF *WHY WE GET FAT*, WROTE IN *THE NEW YORK TIMES*:

> Sugar scares me . . . I'd like to eat it in moderation. I'd certainly like my two sons to be able to eat it in moderation, to not over-consume it, but I don't actually know what that means, and I've been reporting on this subject and studying it for more than a decade. If sugar just makes us fatter, that's one thing. We start gaining weight, we eat less of it. But we are also talking about things we can't see—fatty liver, insulin resistance and all that follows. Officially I'm not supposed to worry because the evidence isn't conclusive, but I do.

I do too!

DO THIS

START MAKING SWAPS IN YOUR KITCHEN.

At this stage you might like to flip to the Getting Equipped section of the book and start getting equipped with some ingredients and staples. (See page 55.)

WHERE'S THE FRUCTOSE?

TABLE SUGAR
50% FRUCTOSE + 50% GLUCOSE

ONE BANANA
**APPROX. 55% SUGAR,
OVER HALF OF WHICH IS FRUCTOSE**

HONEY
40% FRUCTOSE

AGAVE
70–90% FRUCTOSE

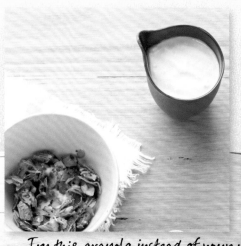

Try this granola instead of your usual.

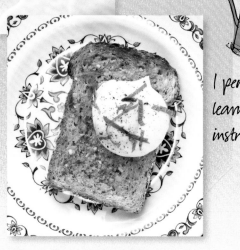

1 Coco-nutty granola

Swap your flakes and sugary granola for this sugar-free version. Makes a great snack, too. Make a big batch to get you through this week! (See recipe on page 76.)

2 "Salted caramel" haloumi and apple

A great one for those of you who need "a little something" after dinner. (See recipe on page 149.)

3 Poached eggs

Swap your usual weekend pancakes or muffin for these lovely little meals. Learn how to make them perfectly, with fun options. (See recipe on page 84.)

I personally think everyone should learn how to poach an egg. See my instructions on page 84.

WEEK 1

2

OPERATION EAT FAT

YES, I'M SUGGESTING YOU EAT FAT.
I know it's unconventional, but it works.

Humans aren't designed to restrict their intake of food. When we fast, our obedient little bodies are programmed to think we're in famine or in a state of emergency, and thus particular hormones and urges kick in to ensure our survival.

When our bodies are deprived of food, our:

▶ survival instinct kicks in and we become obsessed with seeking out food.

▶ systems store any calories ingested for safe-keeping.

And that's why extreme diets don't work. Actually, they're counterproductive. More than 95% cause you to put on weight. Which is why I found this interim phase so important when quitting sugar.

WE HAVE TO REPLACE WHAT WE'RE TAKING OUT.

For both psychological reasons (so we don't get depressed and frustrated from the deprivation) and for physiological reasons (so our bodies don't go into famine mode).

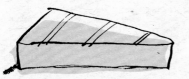

IQS MANTRA 2

REPLACE SUGAR WITH FAT.

You know what? It's this very trick that makes my sugar-quitting program work. I know it might be a bit tough to take at first. But hear me out.

DO THIS

EAT FAT AND PROTEIN.

Once we take out sugar, the best thing you can do is replace it with fat and some protein. I'm talking wholesome, unprocessed fats and quality protein, like eggs, cheese, nuts and coconuts.

The reason is two-fold:

▶ It takes care of the craving for a "treat"—which is part of the sugar addiction. When I replaced my afternoon chocolate treat with a fatty, protein-rich food, I didn't feel like I was denying myself—emotionally or physically.

▶ Fat and protein fill us up. They curb the cravings.

Some white-coat facts to arm yourself with:

1 FAT DOESN'T MAKE YOU FAT (SUGAR DOES).

Eating fat is bad! Right? Actually, no. And this is something we need to get clear on . . .

THE "FAT MAKES US FAT AND SICK" ARGUMENT IS FLAWED.

We all grew up being told fat is bad. On the food pyramid we were all fed at school, fat took up a tiny tip of the iceberg. Saturated fat, we were told, was particularly evil—it led to heart attacks and cholesterol issues.

This thinking can be linked to a study American scientist Ancel Keys conducted in the 1950s and '60s that focused on 22 countries around the world. At the time, incidences of heart disease had increased dramatically in the US and there was pressure to find "the reason," not least because the president at the time had had a near-fatal heart attack. Keys' study found that folk around the world who ate lots of saturated fats (animal and coconut fats) had higher rates of heart disease and cholesterol issues.

BINGO! A REASON!

And so the anti-saturated-fat campaign was launched.

The FDA developed their guidelines based around this messaging (which led to the food pyramid taught to kids around the world) and the low-fat industry was launched. We were told to eat margarine and use so-called vegetable oils, such as canola, corn and soy.

Problem was, the science was faulty.

Keys only ever published the results of seven of the 22 countries. The results of the other 15 countries disproved the theory.

Nutritionists and commentators have only just realized this to be the case and are starting to reassess guidelines. They're realizing the reason that they were after—the common culprit—was actually sugar.

You might find this interesting, too:

As all this was happening several decades back, the US government had been subsidizing farmers to produce polyunsaturated oils (canola, soy and corn) but now had a glut of it that they had to make use of. It was a huge problem. They had to offload it. So the low-fat industry heavily promoted these polyunsaturated oils, with low-fat products becoming pumped full of high-fructose corn syrup (HFCS— a corn oil by-product) to enhance flavor and texture.

2 FAT FILLS US UP—SO WE CAN'T GORGE ON IT.

As I mentioned earlier, fats and proteins (and carbs) have corresponding appetite hormones that act as messengers to the brain to control our appetite. You've probably noticed that when you eat cheese or nuts, they get rid of hunger straightaway.

So, all things being equal (i.e., our systems are in balance), we don't get fat from eating fat and protein. Our bodies ensure this. We get full.

Also, fat actually activates your metabolism by synthesizing several important vitamins, includi[ng] vitamin D. Eating (good) fat [can] actually help you lose weig[ht].

3 *BUT,* WE GORGE ON SUGAR. IN FACT, WE'RE DESIGNED TO.

When we eat fructose, our body doesn't notice it in our system. It goes undetected. And so we can eat and eat and eat it, but our bodies don't feel full. Which is why you can drink a jumbo-sized juice or soft drink. Can you imagine drinking that much yogurt? It would be pretty much impossible.

Some say fructose is good because it doesn't cause insulin spikes (as glucose does). You might see agave described as a low-GI sugar alternative. This can actually be a bad thing, in part because insulin is an appetite-control hormone. In fact, be very wary of low-GI claims while you're on the sugar-quitting mission. Fructose is extremely low-GI and the easiest way to make a product qualify as low-GI is to jam it full of fructose.

PLUS, WE'RE PROGRAMMED TO ACTIVELY SEEK OUT AND BINGE ON SUGAR.

Way back when it was so very rare, we had to stock up when we could.

4 SUGAR TURNS DIRECTLY TO FAT.

Just to ensure you were listening: the way fructose is converted to energy in our bodies means that it sidesteps the fat-creation control mechanism in the liver and is converted directly to fatty acids, and then body fat.

5 SUGAR MESSES WITH OUR HORMONE SYSTEMS.

And, in complex ways, leads to cravings and deficiencies. Thus adding to the binge cycles. And so on it goes . . .

EAT THE RIGHT FATS.

There are many mixed, mostly wrong, messages about fat. Many fats are vital. We need fats for immune health, digestion and metabolism. They act as antioxidants and also get rid of heavy metals and toxins in our systems.

▶ **I cook with ghee (clarified butter) and coconut oil.** These are stable, saturated fats that don't change structure at high heat, and both have anti-inflammatory and antifungal properties. Ghee is available in health food stores and Indian specialty shops. Lard is another good option for high-heat cooking and frying (like your grandmother used to use!).

▶ **I cook with butter and olive oil,** but at moderate temperatures only. Avoid these fats for high-heat frying, they aren't as stable as the ones above.

▶ **I pour with olive, walnut and macadamia oils.** These oils are fantastic on salad. (Note: Don't cook with the walnut oil—it should always be kept cool.)

▶ **I embrace animal fat**—I eat chicken skin and bacon fat. Just not excessively. I believe we are meant to eat the whole food. Plus once you allow yourself this fat, you find you get full on it quickly and don't need a lot of it.

▶ **I eat full-fat dairy.** Again, the whole foods argument. When the fat is taken out, a lot of the enzymes that help break down lactose are also taken out. I found that when I swapped to full-fat milk, I had no dairy-based digestion problems.

▶ **I always use organic butter** instead of processed spreads.

▶ **I avoid all polyunsaturated fats** such as canola, safflower, sunflower, soy and corn oils as they are very unstable. I don't touch trans fats (as in deep-fried foods and so on).

TRY THESE REPLACEMENT FAT/ PROTEIN TREATS:

▶ When the afternoon cravings hit, try some **grilled haloumi cheese**. If you have a sandwich press in the office, pop in a few slices and within minutes you have snack-a-licious goodness on a plate. (Haloumi is available in some supermarkets and cheese shops.)

▶ After dinner, try grilling **walnuts** or tossing them in a pan and then sprinkling them on natural yogurt. I sprinkle some cinnamon or vanilla powder on top, too.

▶ At a restaurant, order an extra **calamari** dish after dinner instead of dessert. Or the **cheese platter**, without the grapes and pear slices.

▶ A thick dollop of **macadamia or almond spread** on a rice cake hits the spot if I'm still hungry after lunch. (See recipe on page 64 on how to make your own.)

AND MIX INTO YOUR COOKING:

▶ **Toasted pumpkin seeds** (toast in a pan until they start to pop—about a minute) or use sprouted pumpkin seeds (see page 59). Toss on salads or on top of your oatmeal or yogurt.

▶ **Avocado**. I love it under cheese on toasted sandwiches.

▶ **Play with different oils**. I pour walnut oil (good for dry eyes) on yogurt and dollop the oil on casseroles. Infused extra-virgin olive oils are great on salads.

▶ **Eggs and more eggs**. Toss two through a pumpkin stir-fry. It gives it a great "cheesy" texture. (See my hash meals on pages 130–5.)

▶ **Bacon**. I chop up two strips and add to a hearty lentil and vegetable soup. I use it for a lush flavor hit.

▶ **Goat cheese**. I sprinkle a chunk on top of salad with a glug of olive oil, Greek-style.

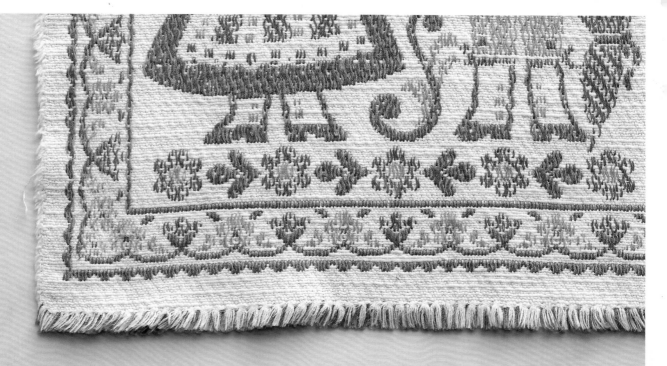

BE CONSCIOUS.

As you switch to this kind of eating, take note of how quickly you feel full, whether your cravings are lessened, whether you feel like you're "missing out on something." I can't stress enough how important it is to witness these kinds of changes. Understanding, as well as having a more intimate relationship with, your internal body will strengthen your resolve over the next few weeks. Find your own way to do this, whether it be through blogging, a morning journal or sharing with your IQS buddy. . . .

KEEP SNACKING.

At least for now. Remember this—if you've been a sugar addict (mild, medium or heavy), you'll probably have some hypoglycemic issues. Which is why you have slumps at 11 a.m. and 4 p.m. I'm betting you've been berating yourself for this, because it generally means you reach for sugar.

Eating regular small meals, 5–6 times a day, is what your body needs for now. In the long-term, once you're off the blood-sugar roller coaster and you've recalibrated, you will find that 2–3 meals a day is best (oh, the time it saves in a day!). But for the next few weeks, when cravings hit, the simple solution is to snack . . . but sugar-free.

My aim when I set out to quit sugar was to get my body back to a balanced state, so I could rediscover my natural appetite mechanisms, instead of reacting from craving to craving.

And ultimately to find my happy weight.

When we're in balance, and eating no sugar, our bodies find a happy homeostasis. And we reach a happy weight. We have few cravings. We get full and genuinely lose interest in food. We burn off the calories in our system. And only then do we feel hungry again when another set of hormones tells the brain we're hungry once more.

This is not some magical state of utopia. It's what our bodies do on their own.

Three recipes to try this week:

1 ### Cheesy biscuits
I promise these will fill you up and satisfy any biscuit/cake fetish. (See page 153.)

2 ### Bacon and egg "cupcakes"
Bake a batch and grab one or two when you get hungry. (See page 88.)

3 ### Sprouted spicy nuts
Try some flavor combinations and up your protein and fat intake in a fun way. (See pages 59 and 146.)

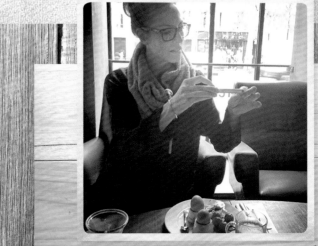

I love sharing my I Quit Sugar food finds on Instagram: sarahwilson.

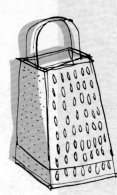

These egg + bacon "cupcakes," are a favorite with my blog readers.

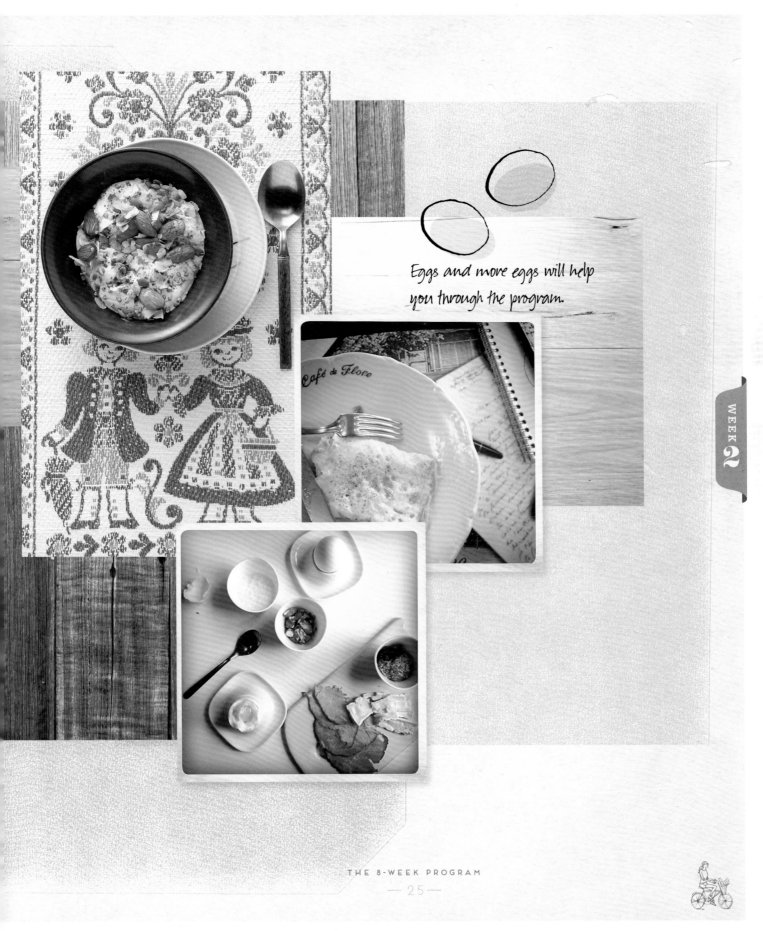

Eggs and more eggs will help you through the program.

HOLD ON TO YOUR SANITY— WE'RE GOING COLD TURKEY!

If you've now cut back on sugar and added good fats into your diet, this won't be as grueling as it sounds. I promise.

Many argue that when you quit sugar, you must quit *all of it . . . for life*. My research found that it was best that all of it goes—in the first instance. Down the track we can lighten up a bit . . . (More on this later.)

During this 8-week program, I found that quitting it all—with no exceptions—was easier. When we allow exceptions, we have to deliberate. If I allow apples, can I also allow pears? If I allow one sugar day a week, should it be Tuesday or Wednesday? Too hard! And likely to lead to a domino-effect of exceptions. Forget that. Do it for real. Life works better when you do.

THERE IS ALSO THIS REASON TO GO COLD TURKEY: YOUR BODY NEEDS TO RECALIBRATE.

You need to find the new set-point. Allowing a little sugar in—some honey here, a bit of fruit there— won't allow your confused system to rid itself of cravings and swings.

DO THIS

GO COLD TURKEY.

From today, the below must go (with no exceptions!):

▶ fresh and dried fruit, fruit juice

▶ granola and granola bars

▶ jams (even if it says no added sugar)

▶ condiments containing sugar, particularly tomato and barbeque sauces, balsamic vinegar

▶ flavored yogurts

▶ honey

▶ agave

▶ palm and coconut sugar

▶ chocolate, soft drinks, etc.

LEARN HOW TO READ FOOD LABELS.

To properly quit sugar, you need to be aware of hidden sugars, to ensure you're keeping to 6 to 9 teaspoons or less of the stuff a day. Take time to pause in the super-market aisle and read the Nutrition Facts labels. Make smart choices by comparing sugar content. On labels, where it says "sugars," it's referring to all sugar and doesn't distinguish fructose-containing sugars. Different sugars contain different amounts of fructose.

For example, table sugar is 50% glucose and 50% fructose, while the sugar in milk is lactose and contains no fructose.

Labels also fail to distinguish added sugar (something many doctors and experts are campaigning to change). So, it can be confusing.

Q ARE ALL VEGGIES CONSIDERED OK? I DID THE MATH AND MY PACK OF SUN-DRIED TOMATOES IS MORE THAN 25% SUGAR!

A Fresh tomatoes are about 5 g of sugar per tomato, so about 1.5 teaspoons. A few slices on a sandwich are fine. But the dried tomatoes are just like any other dried fruit. Drying them concentrates the sugar and gives you a big sugar hit without the asso-ciated bulk that would slow you down if you were eating the whole fruit. We should try to avoid all dried fruits (even ones we think of as savory).

What's more, in the U.S., labels do not provide a "per 100g" or "per 100ml" value, which makes it really difficult to get a picture of the percentage of sugar in a product (see the next page for how to calculate it yourself). In Europe and Australia they provide this amount clearly on the packaging. Again, confusing!

Oh, and the Food & Drug Administration does not require that manufacturers provide a % Daily Value amount for sugar (nor trans fat) because it hasn't yet agreed on a recommended daily requirement. The FDA has devoted pages on its website trying to explain the label-reading process to consumers, and label reading is so un-user-friendly that the packaged food industry took the matter into its own hands a few years ago and launched the Facts Up Front information on the front of their packages . . . prompting the FDA to commit to overhaul-ing the whole system. This has yet to happen.

In the meantime, here are some label-reading guide-lines that work for me:

▷ If sugar is the first or second ingredient, there's a big issue. Labels always list things with the ingredient used most, first.

▷ Look out for other sugars in the list or ingredients: corn syrup, high-fructose corn syrup (hcfs), evapo-rated cane juice, agave, fruit pulp, fruit puree, fruit juice/fruit juice concentrate, blackstrap molasses, diastase, treacle, panocha, sorghum syrup, as well as the "-oses" (sucrose, galactose, maltose, dextrose, etc.), honey, and maple syrup. Brown rice syrup is okay.

▷ With dairy, the first 11 g of sugar per cup, or 4.7g/100g, listed will be lactose (or fructose). Anything on top of that is added sugar.

▷ Drink liquids that contain no sugar. Always. This is because servings are so large; remember a standard can of soda (12 ounces) contains 10 teaspoons of sugar.

To learn how to dissect a Nutrition Facts label more closely, turn the page.

Step 2. Check the serving size.

Now look at the number of servings at the top of the label and assess whether you're likely to eat more or less than this. If you're likely to drink the whole carton of juice, for example, but the servings per carton is 2, you'll need to double the amount of sugar.

Step 1. Find out how many teaspoons of sugar are in a serving:

Scan down the label to the "sugars" (it's often under "total carbohydrates"). The amount is provided in metric quantities—grams or mls. Divide this figure by 4.2 to find out the number of teaspoons of sugar you're consuming in a serving. This serving of yogurt contains 10.5 teaspoons of sugar.

Fruit Yogurt

Nutrition Facts

Serving Size 1 Container (227g)

Amount Per Serving

Calories 240	Calories from Fat 25

	% Daily Value*
Total Fat 3g	4%
Saturated Fat 1.5g	9%
Trans Fat 0g	
Cholesterol 15mg	5%
Sodium 140mg	6%
Total Carbohydrate 46g	15%
Dietary Fiber less than 1g	3%
Sugars 44g	

Protein 9g

Vitamin A	2%	●	Vitamin C	4%
Calcium	35%	●	Iron	0%

*Percent Daily Values are based on a 2,000 – calorie diet. Your daily values may be higher or lower depending on your calorie needs.

You can disregard the % Daily value information, as no daily reference value has been established for sugars because no recommendations have been made for the total amount to eat in a day.

When you're looking at a dairy label, remember the first 11g per cup or 4.7g/100g is lactose. Lactose is fine to consume but anything on top of the 4.7g/100g is added sugar. In this yogurt there's 14.6g of added sugar per 100g (14.6%). This is the best figure to work with when making your calculations.

Step 3. Calculate the percentage of sugar:

To calculate the percentage of sugar in the food, divide the sugar weight by the total weight and then multiply by 100 to calculate the percentage of sugar in a product. This yogurt has 19.3g of sugar per 100g (19.3%). If your chocolate comes out at 46%, then it's almost one-half sugar. Visualize this!!

THE BIG SAUCE SWAP

TAKE A CLOSE-UP OF YOUR CONDIMENTS AND MAKE SOME NEW CHOICES.
HERE ARE SOME SIMPLE SWAPS TO CONSIDER:

Reduced-fat sauces and spreads can contain double the amount of sugar.
Or, in the case of mayonnaise, ten times as much!

FAT-FREE MAYO — **23% sugar** ⟷ **2.2% sugar** — WHOLE EGG MAYO

THE LOW-FAT DAIRY DOOZY

A small tub of "diet" yogurt can often contain up to 6 teaspoons of sugar, even the ones that say "no added sugar." Natural, full-fat yogurt is about 4.7 % (11 g per cup) sugar. But the sugar is lactose, which is fructose-free. Anything over 4.7 % is added sugar.

LOW-FAT YOGURT — **15% sugar** ⟷ **4.7% sugar** — NATURAL YOGURT

Instead of barbeque sauce (54% sugar), use mustard (less than 1% sugar).

BARBEQUE SAUCE — **54% sugar** ⟷ **<1% sugar** — MUSTARD

Instead of balsamic (16% sugar), use apple cider vinegar (less than 1% sugar).

BALSAMIC VINEGAR — **16% sugar** ⟷ **<1% sugar** — APPLE CIDER VINEGAR

Instead of sweet chili sauce (42% sugar), use tamari (less than 1% sugar).

SWEET CHILI SAUCE — **42% sugar** ⟷ **<1% sugar** — TAMARI

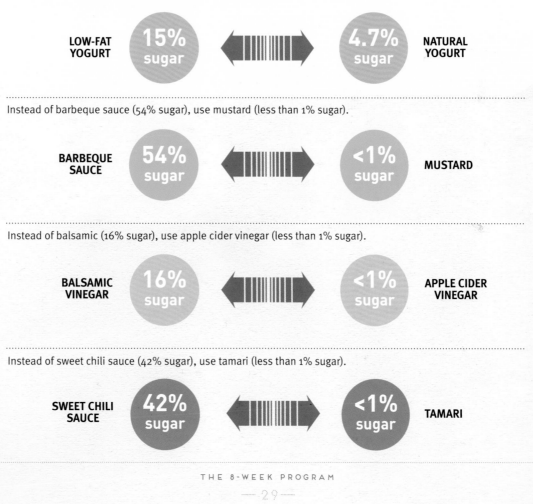

EAT OUT DIFFERENTLY.

Eating out doesn't need to be avoided during these first eight weeks. You just need to be mindful of possible hidden sugars, and try to avoid even glancing at the dessert menu. . . .

▶ Look out for and avoid "honey-roasted," "caramelized" and "balsamic reduction" on menus.

▶ Steer clear of Thai food—the stuff is drenched in palm sugar. I learned this the hard way. I forced myself to eat a stir-fry, vaguely aware it was full of sugar . . . I had a stomachache all night.

▶ Greek cuisine is great and so is pub fare—steak, fries, veggies or fish of the day.

▶ Be wary of tapas and finger food—they often get slathered in more sauces than a main-course dish.

▶ At delis, build your own sandwich rather than grab the pre-made kind so you can choose the spreads yourself.

▶ Similarly, at buffets, opt for dishes with the least amount of ingredients, particularly sauces. So go for the roast dinner, rather than the pasta with the rich tomato sauce.

▶ Ask for olive oil and lemon over salad, or ask for dressing on the side if you're not sure what it comes with. Salads are perilous: they often come drenched in balsamic or, worse, Thousand Island dressing.

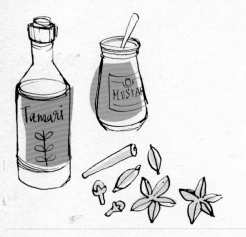

Q WHAT ABOUT ALCOHOL?

A You've possibly been scanning the pages looking for this bit . . . Good news!

WINE, BEER AND PURE SPIRITS CONTAIN MINIMAL FRUCTOSE.

This is because the fructose in the fruit used is converted to alcohol. The drier the wine, the better (so don't touch fortified and dessert wines). But this isn't a license to get drunk. Alcohol has its own fat metabolism and health issues, and is also addictive. Once you've cut out sugar you'll possibly find your tolerance is lower. One or two drinks maximum in one sitting is best.

BEWARE

TONIC WATER IS BRIMMING WITH SUGAR. USE ONLY SELTZER AS A MIXER!

Q IS HFCS (HIGH-FRUCTOSE CORN SYRUP) WORSE OR BETTER THAN SUGAR?

A The short answer—it's on par with sugar in terms of fructose content (about 55%). However (long answer), in the 1980s the US government subsidized corn producers and so the food industry went into overdrive to use up this cheap, new, bountiful product and it flooded the market and our diet. Not surprisingly everyone was told it was healthier than sugar. More recently, though, it's been blamed for the obesity epidemic and stamped as "evil," and cane sugar is now being branded as the healthier alternative. Confused? Don't be. They're both as bad as each other.

START EATING FROM THE "NINE C'S OF GOODNESS"

I FOUND THAT THERE WERE CERTAIN FOODS THAT HELPED ME THROUGH THE FIRST 8 WEEKS.

These were high-protein or high-fat foods, or foods that picked me up in some way.
They all happened to start with "c," funnily enough.

Cacao—You can buy raw cacao nibs at health food shops. They're pure, raw cocoa—an amazing anti-oxidant that gives you an intense chocolate hit.

Chai—Oh, yes. Chai tea. The ritual of heating the milk and adding cardamom, cinnamon bark, ginger and licorice, then pouring cup after cup into a nice glass, makes for very happy times.

Chia—Add these little protein-rich seeds to a smoothie or your yogurt in the morning. They fill you up and do wonders for your digestion.

Cheese—Put a few slices of haloumi in a sandwich press, under the grill or in a pan and eat as an afternoon snack. Or wrap a slice of cheese around a slice of red bell pepper.

Chicken—I keep a bag of shaved chicken or turkey (from the deli at the supermarket) in the fridge and grab a small handful when my energy slumps a few hours before dinner.

Cinnamon—I sprinkle the powder on a variety of foods, like yogurt. I'm also adding cinnamon nibs to my tea. It's great for reducing inflammation, too (for anyone else with autoimmune issues!).

Coconut oil—Very sweet. Add coconut oil to smoothies or cook with it (fry some butternut or kabocha squash in it—it's sublime!). Or just scoop a tablespoon of it straight from the jar. I do!

Coconut water—This stuff is sweet but contains low-to-negligible fructose. It halts sugar cravings in their tracks. The whole baby coconut is best (eat the flesh from it, too!). But the packaged varieties are also good.

Coffee—After I quit sugar I was able to drink coffee again. I'd gone off it for three years because it got my heartbeat too racy. Now I metabolize it just fine. On days I'm missing sweetness in my life, I have it with milk. The lactose is lusciously satisfying.

IQS MANTRA ❸

FIND YOUR BLANK SLATE.

The aim isn't to ban sugar for life. It's to establish a clean canvas from which we can then feel what our bodies need (possibly for the first time in our lives). While sugar is in the system, this is impossible, as we're responding to cravings and highs and lows, not true hunger and need.

IT TAKES ABOUT TWO MONTHS TO FIND
YOUR BLANK SLATE.

After that, it's up to you.

A LITTLE TIP

IF YOU DRINK YOUR COFFEE WITH SUGAR, TRY IT WITH STEVIA. A LOT OF CAFÉS NOW PROVIDE STEVIA PACKETS INSTEAD OF THE NASTIER FAKE SUGARS.

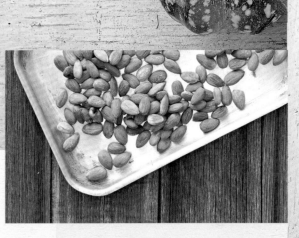

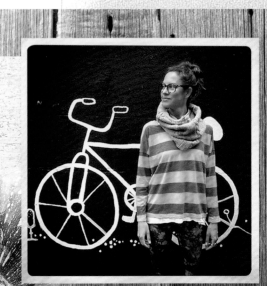

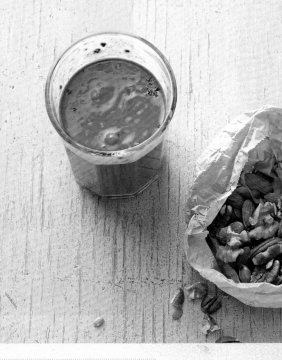

For more snack ideas to make in bulk (like these sprouted almonds and the daikon chips, above), flip to pages 146 and 151.

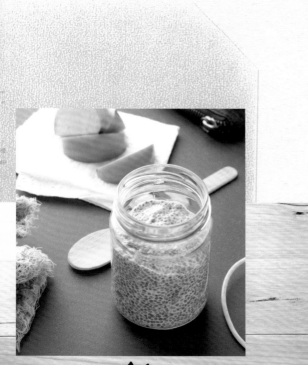
↑ Cashewy chia pudding

1 Make-me-over mojito smoothie

The freshness and coconut-water injection will keep you on track. (See page 112.)

2 Coconut butter

A very nice way to be introduced to coconut. (See page 182.)

3 Cashewy chia puddings

Experiment with these and see how much they fill you up! (See page 80.)

WEEK 3

THE DOUBTS START TO CREEP IN: AM I DOING THE RIGHT THING HERE?
Best, then, to equip yourself with some facts.

Around about this stage I can almost guarantee a little sabotaging voice will pipe up: Why am I putting myself through this pain?

Also—and this is a very bizarre factor—other people will try to sabotage you. Even get angry with you. Everyone I know who has quit sugar has commented on the rough time they get from others. Their efforts are criticized as being misguided. They find themselves defending their diet.

My explanation is this: We all know that sugar is not good for us and we all know, deep down, that we probably eat too much of it. But most people are so attached to it—emotionally and physically—that the idea of not eating it at all petrifies them. Viscerally. I'm betting if we announced we were cutting out peanuts or popcorn, it wouldn't prompt the same ire.

SO WHEN YOU BRAVELY TAKE THE PLUNGE AND QUIT SUGAR, YOU HOLD A MIRROR UP TO OTHERS' FEARS.

You remind them what they wish they could do. And they feel guilty, so then they get angry and lash out.

In the event of such an emergency, here are some comebacks (best issued calmly and without a patronizing sneer).

They say: But sugar is natural!

You say: Indeed it is. But so is petroleum. And arsenic.

As discussed before, our bodies are designed to eat very little fructose. As in a few berries here and there, honey on the rare occasion we stumble upon a hive. The addition of tablespoons (sometimes cups) of sugar to our meals via cereals, sauces and even savory snacks is a very new thing. And not natural. And our bodies have not adjusted to it.

Our digestion and metabolisms haven't changed in 130,000 years. Our sugar intake, however, has. In 150 years, it's gone from o lb. to more than 130 lb. a year.

Yes, sugar is natural. But the amount we're exposed to isn't.

HOW DO I GET MY KIDS TO GO SUGAR-FREE?

I don't have children and I don't yet have an opinion on how (and if) I'd keep all sugar from them so I asked my friends with kids. Their answers and recipes are in the Sugar-Free Kids chapter on page 157.

They say: Cutting fruit out? That's ridiculous!

You say: Fruit contains fructose. And fructose is fructose, no matter the package it comes in.

Yes, whole fruit also contains vitamins and other stuff that's great for us. And indeed the fiber and water in whole fruit diffuses the sugar content. But three things to consider are:

▶ There's little nutritional content in fruit that you can't get from vegetables if you're eating a good variety.

▶ We are designed to metabolize only a small amount of fructose a day, equivalent to two small pieces of fruit, which is what we used to eat prior to the "invention" of sugar in the 1800s. If you're able to eliminate all other sources of fructose (i.e., all hidden sugars added to pasta sauces, bread, etc.), then eating two pieces of fruit is fine. But few of us live like this. At which point you say to your doubter:

> THIS IS WHY I'M CUTTING OUT OTHER SUGAR—
> SO THAT I CAN EAT A LITTLE FRUIT EACH DAY.

(Note: Fruit is introduced toward the end of the 8-week program.)

▶ Also, it really is a very modern thing that we eat so much fruit. Our grandparents didn't eat four pieces a day, as we're told to do these days. And as recently as twenty years ago, fruit juice was a treat, not something you drank from jumbo containers each day.

> P.S. I DON'T THINK FRUIT SHOULD BE DEMONIZED.

Or any food that's legitimately nutritious. I just found it helpful to cut fruit out for two months while my body rebalanced. And to become aware of the fact that it does contain a lot of sugar and that it should be consumed mindfully.

They say: We shouldn't be cutting food out; moderation is the answer!

You say: If only. The problem is, moderation is nearly impossible with sugar. For so many of us it's all or, well, nothing.

Sugar is a drug. We know that sugar interacts with reward systems in the brain in much the same way as addictive drugs. Studies have found rats fed sugar not only became addicted, but when they were denied it for a short period then later exposed to it, they binged on larger quantities of sugar—and other substances like alcohol.

For many of us, a moderate amount of sugar is not achievable because even just a taste of it sets off a desire for more. Much more. I personally can't eat one chocolate chip cookie. I'm not that person. I'm more like Miranda in that scene in *Sex and the City* where she has to put the cake in the trash and then douse it with water so she won't eat more. I get the taste and I keep going.

Not everyone's like this. But I am.

If my comebacks fail, then there's always this (for your own personal comfort):

> **All truth passes through three stages. First, it is ridiculed. Second, it is violently opposed. Third, it is accepted as being self-evident.** —ARTHUR SCHOPENHAUER

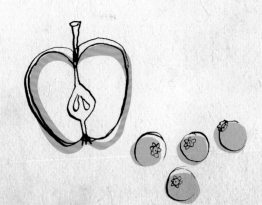

WALK AWAY FROM THE FRUIT JUICE.

A glass of apple juice (freshly squeezed or otherwise) contains the same amount of sugar (fructose) as a glass of Coke, which is about 10–12 teaspoons.

And know this: when sugar is in liquid form—soft drink or juice—the fructose and glucose hit the liver faster. The speed with which the liver has to do its work means the liver will convert much of the sugar in the drink to fat, inducing insulin resistance. And so on.

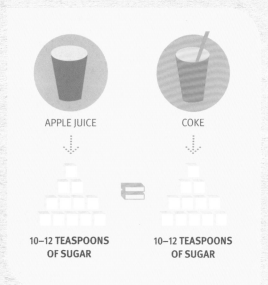

APPLE JUICE   COKE

10–12 **TEASPOONS** OF SUGAR   10–12 **TEASPOONS** OF SUGAR

CALCULATE HOW MUCH SUGAR YOU ARE ACTUALLY EATING.

Now's a really good time in the journey to remind yourself how much white stuff you were consuming before you quit. Had you been kidding yourself . . . even just a little? I had. So I sat down with pen and paper and added up the exact number of teaspoons of the stuff I had been eating. It was shocking. I suggest you try the same exercise. It's a good reminder of why you're doing this.

1. On the food label, scan down to "sugars" (in gs or mls).

2. Divide that number by 4.2 (round down to 4 if you don't have a calculator) to get the number of teaspoons.

3. Remember to subtract the first 11 g per cup of sugar in dairy products (which is lactose). And if the serving size is ½ cup, for example, adjust and subtract 5.5 g.

4. Double or triple the serving amount if you tend to eat more, as I do. Be realistic!

SOME EXTRA CONSIDERATIONS:

- When calculating sugar in a piece of fruit, it gets tricky. But to give an indication, an apple is about 2–3 teaspoons of sugar (more than half of which is fructose, so it's almost the equivalent of 4.5 teaspoons of sugar); a banana is about 4 teaspoons of sugar.

- That handful of raisins or dates on your granola? About 5–7 teaspoons. Dates and raisins are almost 70% sugar!

AT A GLANCE:

A glass of fruit juice = 8–12 teaspoons.

Cinnamon raisin toast = 6–7 teaspoons per serving (two pieces).

A fruit muffin = up to 11 teaspoons.

A dollop of ketchup = 1–2 teaspoons.

Kellogg's Just Right cereal = 4–8 teaspoons (depending on serving size).

A small tub of low-fat yogurt = up to 6 teaspoons.

A serving of pasta sauce (from a jar) = about 4 teaspoons.

Jot down a typical day's worth and add it all up.

What did you arrive at?

AND REMEMBER:

FROM A BIOLOGICAL POINT OF VIEW, WE'RE ONLY DESIGNED TO BE ABLE TO HANDLE THE SUGAR CONTAINED IN TWO PIECES OF FRUIT IN A DAY: 5–6 TEASPOONS.

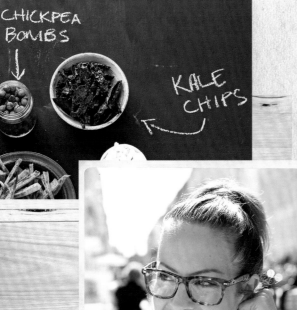

1 Zucchini "cheesecake"

A simple, fun dish that proves you don't need to eat sugar and carbs for breakfast. (See page 96.)

2 Kale chips

A quick snack that's so much better than an afternoon muffin. (See page 151.)

3 Rooibos chai

Sweet and special, for when the Doubting Thomas voices in your head are really getting to you. (See page 117.)

WEEK 4

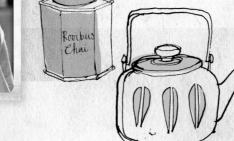

YOU'RE ALMOST HALFWAY!

Stick with things. And once fructose is out of your system, your body will start to tell you whether it wants to eat fruit—or is happy with vegetables instead—and how much it wants. It will stop bingeing.

Your body will seek balance and will find it if it's not interfered with.

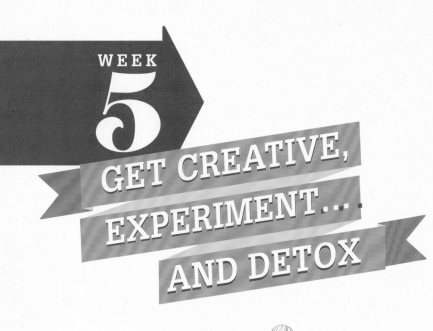

WEEK 5
GET CREATIVE, EXPERIMENT... AND DETOX

CRAVINGS— THEY'RE UGLY AND DISPIRITING.
But they're normal so it's important to keep going.

As I said at the outset, studies show it takes 21–28 days to break a habit. Another study says it takes 66 days, but that it doesn't matter if you lapse, so long as your intention is to continue.

I like this thinking. It acknowledges how we humans operate. Each day we stay off sugar, we're creating new habits in our cells, our hormones and in our brains.

LIKE A MUSCLE, THE MORE WE PRACTICE, THE MORE THIS WAY OF BEING BECOMES SECOND NATURE.

But if you do lapse—say you sneak honey in your tea or pick at a friend's birthday cake—don't fret and don't give up. It's fine. Just keep your intention on track.

Tomorrow is a new day.

DO THIS

DISTRACT YOURSELF WITH ALTERNATIVE SWEETNESS.

Often sugar is simply a treat. A punctuation point in the day, a reward for completing something challenging, or a tool to get you through a difficult task. I know I used to reach for sugar when I was working—it made the task feel less onerous and took the edge off so I didn't resent doing it.

Plan out a few activities that can take the place of the comfort drawn from sugar. Cutting emotional attachment is a huge part of this process. It's been the hardest part for me.

I found changing a few lifestyle habits really helped. I sat down and wrote out all the moments that were going to feel hard while quitting sugar. And then matched it with a fix. I really suggest doing the same. It's illuminating. And necessary.

➡ *Try these tricks on the opposite page.*

MY SWEET DISTRACTIONS

CHALLENGING MOMENT	THE FIX
Mid-morning empty feeling or agitation (especially in the face of a difficult task)	I find eating breakfast a little later helps. I push it back so it coincides with my "snack attack." This might not work for anyone who's desperately hungry when they wake.
Afternoon slump	I assign chores that require a walk, such as a visit to the post office, or I stroll to the park for some fresh air. When I'm wanting to indulge, I'll buy a new flavor of tea—green, chai, herbal. I've invested in a gorgeous pot, which makes the tea ritual all the more "treaty."
Coffee with friends who tend to order biscuits or cakes	I order a very large pot of chai to fill me up. The tea-straining ritual also distracts me nicely. Or I suggest a catch-up over a walk instead.
Plane rides	I buy nuts at the airport to take on board. Or I bring my own from home.
When I'm in the middle of a tricky project	Previously, writing a long paper or cranking out a complicated email would lead me to the pantry for an anxiety fix. Now, I get up and burn sandalwood incense sticks or cinnamon bark oil. The woodiness and sweetness smells almost as smooth and velvety as chocolate. Then I make a pot of green tea.
After dinner	I often seek something sweet around 8 p.m. Now I try these alternatives:

I often seek something sweet around 8 p.m. Now I try these alternatives:

▶ **Cheese.** It's decadent and it fills me up immediately. Faster than nuts, I find.

▶ **Have a bath and read a book.** Sweetness in another shape!

▶ **Brush my teeth** after dinner.

PAUSE FOR 20 MINUTES.

When in the clutches of a craving, simply tell yourself: Let's wait 20 minutes.

Only 20 minutes. And then see if you still need a sweet fix. In the meantime, make a cup of tea. Again, pause and take note of how the craving shifts.

THIS PAUSING AND LOOKING IS IMPORTANT—IT BUILDS THE "I CAN DO THIS" MUSCLE, MAKING IT EASIER NEXT TIME.

START TO DETOX.

Some of you, around about now, will be nauseous, dizzy, constipated, have aching kidneys and joints. This means that you're withdrawing and detoxing.

And it's a good sign.

Your body is ejecting toxins from your fat cells and they're swirling around your system on their way out. But they're definitely on their way out!

IQS MANTRA 4

CROWDING OUT

This is a theory I subscribe to with my eating overall. Rather than engage in prohibitive, restrictive eating ("I must quit chocolate," "I have to stop eating muffins"), swap tactics.

EAT MORE OF THE GOOD STUFF.

Each meal, load up on vegetables, nuts, seeds, legumes, healthy grains, etc., and "crowd out" the "bad food." Stuff yourself with spinach and you'll be too full to eat any chocolate!

THERE ARE THINGS YOU CAN DO TO FEEL BETTER AND SPEED THINGS UP:

▶ **Drink lots of warm water** (herbal tea is good) to flush the toxins out.

▶ **Get acupuncture.** It can help with cravings, withdrawal and toxin flushing.

▶ **Visit a sauna,** and sweat things out.

▶ **Take digestive-care and bowel-movement helpers.** You might like to try slippery elm powder (see Resources, page 205) and chia seeds—both are quite mild and won't clog you up but you will have to drink extra water to ensure they do their job well. I also take good-digestive-bacteria supplements: acidophilus tablets/powders, green powders and chlorophyll. But not all at once. I alternate.

▶ **Try some herbal supplements.** Here's a few that have worked for me, but I very much recommend visiting a qualified naturopath or herbalist before you start experimenting.

Calcium and magnesium. Best taken in a formula together, I was told. Magnesium and calcium help combat adrenal stress, curb sugar desire and protect against metabolic syndrome.

Gymnema. A traditional Ayurvedic Indian herb, which powerfully curbs sugar cravings by balancing the release of insulin from the pancreas. (See Resources, page 205). Chromium (200 mg daily) is also good for regulating insulin.

Green tea. Green tea reduces the glycemic index of food intake (so best to drink it just before meals).

Cinnamon (1 teaspoon per day). Helps control blood sugar levels and stops sugar cravings. Easy to add to breakfast or a hot drink, such as chai tea.

Licorice root tea. Tastes sweet without containing sugar. Supports healthy, strong adrenal glands and helps combat stress. When stress is under control, you'll crave sugar less.

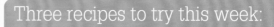

Three recipes to try this week:

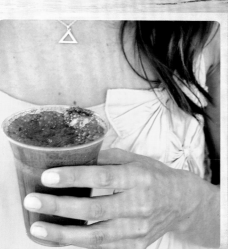

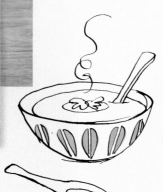

↑ I drink green drinks whenever I feel the cravings start up.

1 **Sweet green meal-in-a-tumbler**
Kick your day off with one of these and you'll be crowding out all temptations. (See page 110.)

2 **Cheesy green mish-mash soup**
A complete detox helper. Perfect at the end of the day. (See page 129.)

3 **Cooling avocado soup**
Green, refreshing and zesty. (See page 138.)

WEEK 6
ADD SOME SWEETNESS BACK IN

I'M NOT TALKING SUGAR, HERE. I'M TALKING ABOUT SWEET FLAVORS. After about six weeks, most of you will find you're no longer craving sugar, or sweetness.

Now is a good time to start playing a little with some sweet-orientated ingredients: some low-fructose vegetables and fruits, some safe sugar substitutes and some other spices and flavors.

But all sweeteners—fructose-tainted or otherwise—should be used in moderation. Research suggests over-use of artificial sweeteners might contribute to weight gain. It can cause sugar cravings, meaning you'll seek out calories from other sweet sources. (Also see "Beware," opposite.)

Our brains expect sweetness to be accompanied by corresponding calorie density, and when it's not, we're thrown off kilter. This causes us to seek out calories from other sources, and we overeat.

DO THIS

ADD A SMALL AMOUNT OF FRUIT.

At this stage in the game, it's best just to try a little of the low-fructose fruit. For your records:

▶ **Low-fructose fruit:** kiwis, grapefruit, honeydew melon, blueberries and raspberries.

▶ **Medium-fructose fruit:** mandarins, plums, peaches, strawberries and oranges.

▶ **High-fructose fruit:** grapes, cherries, apples, mangoes and bananas. Avoid these!

Q I LOVE BAKING SO HOW DO I SWAP OUT SUGAR IN MUFFINS AND CAKES WITH SOMETHING ELSE?

A You can replace with glucose (dextrose), brown rice syrup or stevia granules (or drops). Dextrose is a bit tricky, as it weighs about half as much as sugar, but takes up more fluid, so you'll need to play around with it. Stevia in the granulated form can be used exactly like sugar, although I tend to put in a little less as I find stevia sweeter-tasting (others don't). Brown rice syrup works best where you've been instructed to use honey. (For conversion details see page 66.)

FAKING IT:
THE SAFE SUGAR ALTERNATIVES

Everyone likes to slap on a "no added sugar" label. Health food shops are some of the worst for this. But read labels carefully. Agave, maple syrup, honey, fruit juice extract, molasses, corn syrup—they're all fructose.

There are many fake sugars out there, most of which I wouldn't feed to a potted plant.

After a full year of researching the options, I choose to work with the first two, mostly safe, sweeteners below. Please note that throughout this book I've tended to steer my recipes toward the less sweet end of the spectrum. Once you quit sugar, your sensitivity to sweetness is more acute, so you need less to get your kick (also see my warning below).

BROWN RICE SYRUP (sometimes called "rice syrup" or "rice malt syrup") is a natural sweetener that is made from fermented cooked rice and is a blend of complex carbohydrates, maltose and glucose. It's a relatively slow-releasing sweetener so it doesn't dump on the liver as much as pure glucose or sucrose does. Make sure the ingredients list only rice (and water). Some versions add extra (fructose-containing) sugars. You can find brown rice syrup in health food stores and some supermarkets.

STEVIA is made from stevioside (which is 300 times sweeter than sugar) and rebaudioside (450 times sweeter than sugar). It comes as a liquid or mixed with erythritol to form granules (be sure to read the label as the liquid is more potent than regular sugar; the granules can be substituted one-for one). Stevia is a natural alternative, derived from a leaf and contains no fructose. Most researchers deem it safe but still don't really know what the human body does with the stevia once ingested.

OTHER SWEETENERS that are okay to use in moderation: xylitol (a sugar alcohol extracted from birch cellulose that can be digested by our bodies—most can't—and that has antibacterial properties), glucose syrup (or maltodextrin or maltodextrose, not to be confused with maltitol) and dextrose (100% glucose; bought as a powder), all of which can be found in the baking section of some supermarkets, or in health food shops or online (see Resources, page 205).

THE REST: don't touch. Most have been shown to be either carcinogenic or entirely indigestible, thus causing myriad health issues (um, ever noticed how "sugar-free" gum can make you loose-boweled and gassy?!). Many of the fake sugars available are banned in parts of Europe, deemed unsafe. Enough said.

BEWARE: Even non-fructose sugars, such as glucose, are not good to eat in large quantities and will cause insulin wobbliness too, albeit in a far more manageable way. What's more, studies at the University of Washington have found that consuming *any* kind of sweetener—even the "fake" ones that don't contain sugar as such—can cause a blood sugar spike and continue a sugar addiction. Just the sweet taste can trigger insulin and metabolic responses. Eat "sweet" treats as treats only! Even when a recipe contains a safe sweetener, it should be eaten with care. And not without other nutrients and fiber, not in large quantities, and preferably not every day, unless the recipe is sweetened with coconut oil, coconut flesh, coconut cream or coconut milk only.

DO THIS

ADD IN A FEW FUN FLAVORS.

▶ **Vanilla powder**—sprinkled on yogurt.

▶ **Cinnamon**—instead of sugar in your coffee. Try adding a dash of it to coffee as it brews.

▶ **Licorice root**—in baked things. A small teaspoon of the root adds instant sweetness.

▶ **Almond milk**—add it to tea as well as smoothies.

▶ **Sautéed onion**—to sweeten pasta sauces. Many savory foods have sugar added. This is especially true for foods with a tomato base due to tomatoes' acidity. Sweeten with lots of cooked onion instead. Let the onion caramelize on the stove top until it's deeply golden, the sugar oozing out.

▶ **Roast vegetables**—instead of dessert. Eat the roasted veggies at the end of the meal and you will feel far less in need of a sweet. The most dessert-like ones are sweet potato, squash, beets and carrots.

▶ **Sweet sugar-free drinks**—licorice root tea, chai tea, milk sprinkled with coffee, and herbal teas that contain roasted dandelion root (tastes like coffee/chocolate), licorice, cinnamon, chili, maca, ginger or cardamom. And, of course, coconut water.

TIP

WHEN BUYING SOY, ALMOND OR RICE MILK, BE SURE TO CHECK WHETHER IT HAS ADDED SUGAR. SOME CONTAIN MORE THAN 2 TEASPOONS PER GLASS. (OR SEE PAGE 65 FOR MY EASY HOMEMADE ALMOND MILK RECIPE.)

THE DEAL WITH CHOCOLATE . . .

The most common question I get asked is: What about sugar-free chocolate? Well, so far there are very few commercial versions on the market using safe fructose-free sweeteners; good options include Frusano's, Lucienne's, Dante Confections and Coco Polo.

Here are some suggestions for getting your chocolate fix:

▶ A small handful of raw cacao nibs.

▶ Make your own, using coconut oil and raw cacao powder. (See page 177 for my recipe.)

▶ Try one of the 99% or 100% cacao versions from specialty chocolate shops, although they are very bitter. I also think the 85% cocoa varieties are OK once you've been off sugar a few months. You'll need to limit yourself to just a few squares—and you'll need to be "clean" to have such discipline.

▶ And, of course, there are plenty of sugar-free chocolate recipes featured later in the book.

BEWARE

▶ SURE, 70% COCOA DARK CHOCOLATE IS BETTER THAN MILK CHOCOLATE, BUT IT STILL CONTAINS ALMOST 30% SUGAR. DO THE MATH: A 50 G SERVING CONTAINS 15 G, OR ALMOST 4 TEASPOONS, OF SUGAR.

▶ SOME "SUGAR-FREE" CHOCOLATE CONTAINS AGAVE, WHICH IS UP TO 90% FRUCTOSE.

▶ SOME "SUGAR-FREE" CHOCOLATES ARE SWEETENED WITH MALTITOL, WHICH IS ONE OF THE COMMON SUGAR ALCOHOLS. OUR BODIES CAN'T INGEST MORE THAN A HALF TO TWO-THIRDS OF ANY SUGAR ALCOHOL. SO, WHAT DOESN'T GET INGESTED PROPERLY INTO YOUR BLOODSTREAM FEEDS THE BACTERIA IN YOUR LARGE INTESTINE. NOT NICE.

1 My raspberry ripple

Finally, some chocolate, but without the angst and sugar crashes. (See page 186.)

2 Coconut fluffs with spiced berry swirl

A very treaty breakfast! (See pages 98 and 100.)

3 Crunchy-nut cheesecake

For when it's time to indulge and impress your friends with a classic "sweet" treat. (See page 191.)

WEEK 6

Want to know which skillet to buy? Flip to my tips on page 57.

RECOVERING FROM LAPSES

AROUND ABOUT NOW, THINGS BECOME A LITTLE EASIER.

I've found most people are over the detox period and the withdrawal, and are in the glorious swing of things.

At this stage it can be tempting to relax, to be a little too proud of yourself. And you lapse.

So, you have to be careful. I've lapsed. Many times. But each time I've been aware of it and—here's the thing—allowed it. Which has enabled me to remain mature about whether I actually enjoyed sugar at all.

I find I lapse not when I'm around fully sugared foods but when I'm exposed to "sort of healthy" foods. Like dark chocolate strawberries, or a gluten-free muffin sweetened with organic maple syrup. This is because the issue becomes one of degree. I've had to become aware of this.

But to be honest, if I find myself eating these "healthy" sugared foods occasionally, I just go with it. I don't punish myself. I can revert to my blank slate pretty quickly by eating some fat and crowding out with lots of greens. I find it's helpful to reflect and correct once the moment is gone. Then I can choose. Do I want to continue eating this? Or do I want to be clean and

clear? It doesn't have to be a big deal and I can move on from it.

I know some other sugar-free converts can't operate like this. You will only know where you're at once you have sugar out of your system.

Lapses have served as great reminders of why I quit.

When I have sugar I can witness how my body isn't sated by sugar but wants MORE. It's a little scary. And so I have to move forward with a bit of care.

GENTLE AND KIND.

I actually recommend—after being sugar-free for a good two months—testing yourself. Have a chocolate chip cookie. Monitor your enjoyment and reaction to it.

It's been one of the most liberating things for me— to see how measured and grounded I can be with it. Only a few short months ago, sugar controlled me. Now I can witness what it does to my body with curiosity. And decide to leave it alone.

This is freedom.

TRY THESE LAPSE FIXERS:

▶ During or just after a lapse, pause and take note. How do you find the smell? The taste? Can you feel yourself wanting to reach for more? How did you feel afterward? Each time I was amazed how much I was repulsed by the taste; it seemed so acidic and cloying.

▶ Next, move. Walk, swim, do a yoga class, sweat a little. Literally move on from it.

▶ Eat some densely nutritious food—protein, fats and vegetables only. Avoid starchy carbs for a day (they'll just add to the blood-sugar load). I find warm food—not salads—work best. You want to "ground" yourself again; warm, heavy foods are best for this. I'll buy a piece of fish and grill it with some steamed vegetables with lots of butter. Or I'll buy a hamburger with cheese. And bacon. But hold the fries and bun.

▶ The next day, ensure you don't touch any sugar or stimulants. It only takes half a day to feel on track again. Back off from fruit, tea, coffee, etc.

▶ And most importantly: don't punish yourself. It's no big deal.

When we get harsh, we tend to swing right back into the crave-reward cycle that fuels sugar addiction.

FACT

STUDIES HAVE SHOWN THAT WHEN PEOPLE ACKNOWLEDGE AND FORGIVE THEMSELVES FOR A BAD FOOD CHOICE, THEY'RE BETTER ABLE TO RESIST NEXT TIME.

TIP

LATE-NIGHT CRAVING FIX—BRUSH YOUR TEETH. MOST TOOTHPASTES CONTAIN A SMALL AMOUNT OF SWEETENER (NOTHING WORTH WORRYING ABOUT). AFTER RINSING, DRINK A GLASS OF WATER TO FOOL YOUR STOMACH INTO THINKING YOU'VE CONSUMED SOMETHING SWEET. SPIT IT ALL OUT AGAIN, AN ACTION THAT SYMBOLICALLY "REJECTS" THE SWEETNESS WHILE ALSO STOPPING YOU FROM EATING FURTHER.

Q **IS SUGAR-FREE CHEWING GUM OK?**

A Sugar-free gum contains high-intensity sweeteners (like Ace K, aspartame, alitame and sucralose) and a range of sugar alcohols (like sorbitol, isomalt and mannitol). These sweeteners increase the pH level in your intestines, reduce the amount of good bacteria and can have similar effects as fructose. The sugar alcohols are an issue since our bodies are only able to ingest a fraction of them once in our system. The rest goes into our bloodstream and feeds the bacteria in our large intestine, leading rather delightfully to diarrhea and gas. Which is why so many of these products warn of a "laxative effect." I avoid them. But if you're a gum fan, look out for those sweetened with xylitol only. There are quite a few on the market these days.

WEEK **7**

TRY COCONUT.

Coconut really is going to become your friend, in all its forms—flakes, shavings, oil, cream, milk and, of course, fresh. The stuff is particularly good for cravings and lapses.

Coconut oil is mostly made up of medium-chain fatty acids (MCFAs), which produce a whole host of health benefits. They're small enough to permeate cell membranes easily, do not require special enzymes to be broken down so are easily digested, and they are immediately converted into energy rather than being stored as fat. But unlike carbohydrates, coconut oil does not produce an insulin spike in your bloodstream. This saves you from a slump. Energy, a sense of fullness, a sweet hit and no aftereffects. A quadruple bonus!

If you're lucky enough to come across virgin (young/green) coconuts (they have a white casing, not the brown hard shell of a mature coconut), drink the juice and scrape the flesh out with a spoon to use in smoothies and recipes. To open, either ask the person you bought it from to do so, or invest in a coconut opener.

Coconuts do contain sugar, and it can vary depending on the age (younger coconuts have less sugar). But in unsweetened coconut products, these quantities are quite low (about 2 g per 100 ml), plus the sugar is mostly composed of glucose and a lot less fructose. When reading coconut product labels, be aware that the sugar content is mostly glucose, so it should not be cause for too much alarm.

Here are some coconut ideas to get you started:

▷ **Have a glass of coconut water/juice.** It's three times more hydrating than water, is fat- and (mostly) sugar-free, and is an amazing electrolyte. Go fresh if you can. Otherwise there are some great packaged ones around—look out for versions that are organic, fair-trade and have traveled the least distance. I also choose versions that package the juice straight from the coconut, limiting oxidation. They're a lot sweeter!

▷ **Play around with smoothies.** Add coconut oil (about 1 tablespoon) to your favorite blend (see pages 109–18 for some recipes), replace milk with coconut water, and/or add coconut flesh to the mix to bulk things up beautifully.

▷ **Simply eat a tablespoon or two of coconut oil** straight from the jar. I do this most afternoons to get me through to dinner and to nip a sweet craving in its sneaky little tracks. There is a lot of evidence to show that this daily habit will help you lose weight!

▷ **Toast unsweetened coconut flakes** lightly in a pan and sprinkle on oatmeal or yogurt with some walnuts and cinnamon.

▷ **Pan-fry some kabocha or butternut squash chunks in coconut oil.** Sprinkle with salt (to tenderize the squash) and some cinnamon. Just before serving, stir through some unsweetened coconut flakes or unsweetened shredded coconut and stir until golden. A great little meal or snack on the fly!

▷ **Coconut ice cream!** Simply put a can of coconut cream (not milk, and not a "light" version) in the fridge—it thickens to a soft ice-cream consistency within a few hours.

▷ **Stew fruit in coconut milk** or pour some over strawberries for insta-dessert.

▷ **Make rice pudding with coconut milk.** Simply heat leftover brown rice (or quinoa, or oats) with a good splash of the milk—creamy and sweet! Add cinnamon and nuts.

▷ **Make your own coconut butter** (see page 182) and eat straight from the fridge, or spread on toast or pancakes. (Note: Coconut butter is "pureed" coconut flakes; coconut oil is the more refined oil extracted from the flesh. Some brands confuse "butter" and "oil," just so you know.)

▷ **Add the soft flesh of a fresh coconut** (once you've drunk the juice) to some mashed, stewed pear and serve with good-quality cream.

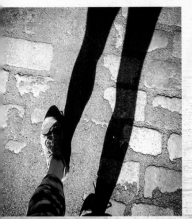

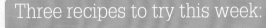

Three recipes to try this week:

1
Fluffy squash and chia muffins
Dense and filling—you'll forget your lapse in no time. (See page 95.)

2
Coconut butter
A simple way to fall in love with coconut. (See page 182.)

3
Sausage, walnut and beet hash
Make yourself a *proper* lunch. This is the best lapse-fixer. (See page 133.)

WEEK 7

BEWARE

THAI FOOD USES A LOT OF COCONUT MILK (GREAT)—BUT A LOT OF PALM SUGAR, TOO . . . STICK WITH INDIAN FOOD INSTEAD.

Coconut products are my secret ↑ weapons for the I Quit Sugar journey.

REFINING
AND MOVING FORWARD

YOU'VE MADE IT!
YOU'VE BROKEN THE CYCLE.
After almost 60 days of repeatedly saying no to sugar, you've built new neural pathways and allowed your body to recalibrate.

When I got to the two-month mark, I remember someone asked me if I missed sugar. Their question was tinged with pity. I answered: "Gosh, I hadn't really thought about it." And this is the sublime point of doing this whole crazy experiment. Soon enough, you wake up and realize sugar is simply not an issue.

When I set out, I wanted to feel clean and clear. But mostly I wanted to be free of sugar. Free from its grip. I wanted to be able to decide how much sugar I needed. In the process, sugar just lost its appeal. As a wonderful consequence. Naturally.

There's an assumption—and I certainly started out this way—that living sugar-free would remain a battle forever. It isn't. The enemy just leaves the battlefield.

I went sugar-free. And I became freed from sugar.

SO WHERE AM I NOW?

It took me eight weeks to get off sugar completely. I followed the steps I outline here in this book. I reduced my intake by making simple swaps. I replaced sugar with fat, and I didn't stay too rigid. I remained gentle, kind, curious and experimental. I ensured my body wasn't left deprived of energy. In fact, I overdid the energy replacements and crowded out the bad stuff with a smorgasbord of densely nutritious and detoxing food. I felt better than I've ever felt, even while going through withdrawal. I was no longer hungry, for the first time in as long as I can remember. I'd arrived at a blank-slate state.

AND MY BODY—AGAIN FOR THE FIRST TIME IN LIVING MEMORY—WAS ABLE TO TELL ME WHAT IT NEEDED, MEAL TO MEAL.

I'm not militant about being sugar-free. If a burger comes with ketchup on top, I let it be. If I realize the curry I'm eating is sweetened, I don't freak out. I eat beets and carrots (which contain a high percentage of sugar, as much as some of the low-fructose fruits) even though some sugar quitters don't. As I said before, I occasionally lapse, too. But only a little. Because I'm able to correct myself easily now. It's not really lapsing. I'm just continuing the experiment.

DO THIS

FIND YOUR OWN WAY.

We're letting go of the training wheels and now you're on your own. But here are some pointers for the road ahead:

▶ **Ask yourself what your approach to sugar is now.** What's your body telling you? It's quite good to do a "so where am I now" rundown this week. Stamp out your stance. Be clear with yourself.

▶ **But keep testing and being curious.** This will always be an experiment. I advise enjoying the ride, allowing for lapses and corrections.

▶ **Keep informed and engaged.** I find staying up-to-date on the latest science and developments in regards to sugar very helpful. It helps to remind me of why I'm doing the experiment. You might like to join the I Quit Sugar communities on iquitsugar.com.

▶ **Don't become an anti-sugar bore.** I had to be conscious of this. There's nothing worse than a reformed smoker/drinker/sugar addict ramming their message down others' throats. Far better to simply "be your message." Live it, radiate it, be an inspiration.

GO EASY ON THE FAT.

I kind of got excited about the "replace sugar with fat" thing for a while when I first quit and had to pull back after a few weeks. This plan isn't a license to pig out! My bet, though, is that by the eighth week your body will tell you how much it needs and you'll settle into a nice rhythm. Mine did, but I continue to eat a lot more (healthy, clean, saturated) fat than I used to.

Q WHAT'S THE DEAL WITH TOOTH-PASTE? IT TASTES SWEET AND I THINK MINE CONTAINS SACCHARIN . . .

A Most toothpastes contain no sugar but a very small amount of saccharin, about 0.2% of the total volume. There are reports linking saccharin to cancer, but at levels equivalent to about 606 standard tubes of toothpaste every day for 50 years. My view: there are other things to worry about.

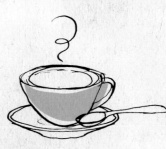

▶ I lost about 9 lb.—not much, but visibly I looked less puffy and I feel like I'm the right weight for my age and height and food quantity choices.

▶ I now have a flat stomach—no more bloating or fluid retention. Seriously. I just don't get it anymore.

▶ I have a clear head and rarely get slumps.

▶ I get full from a meal—happily full.

▶ I don't get "sugar hangovers." I now realize that many of my hangovers after a big dinner were actually from sugar, not always due to alcohol or the late night.

▶ My autoimmune disease is healing—slowly, slowly.

HOW MUCH SUGAR DO I EAT NOW?

I'm not sure exactly. As I say, I'm not militant. I'm not counting out the teaspoons every day as I have a good "gut" feel for what's right for my body. I limit it as much as I can and avoid the prime culprits (dried fruit, juice, sauces etc.—all things I'm happy to live without now that I know they're not benign).

▶ I try to eat products with less than 3–6% of sugar. (See page 27.) Wherever possible.

▶ I eat 1–2 servings of fruit a day. Mostly berries.

▶ I slip in some 85% chocolate and the occasional "sweet treat." (See recipe ideas, page 173.) But they're now treats, not everyday necessities. And besides, I mostly make my own chocolate these days (see page 177).

As I said from the outset, I was simply curious. I started the experiment and kept going. While I feel good, I'll continue to keep going.

I COULD GO BACK TO EATING SUGAR. BUT I DON'T WANT TO.

To all the naysayers out there who freak out about the extremeness of going sugar-free, I say, relax. Since I'm no longer addicted, I'm able to allow a little into my diet.

A little doesn't send me over the edge these days. A little doesn't prevent me from being able to correct. And, the best thing of all, a little is all I feel like.

I'm aware of, and alive to, sugar. So I know where the sugar traps are and I can avoid them.

And this is precisely where I wanted to get to.

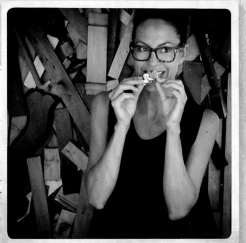

1 Breakfast casserole
Make up a big batch and freeze it in portions so you have some staples for the weeks ahead. (See page 104.)

2 Kale pesto
Make up a big patch of tasty pesto to have on hand for breakfast (on toast, on eggs) or lunch (stir through a salad) or dinner (with zucchini fettuccine). (See page 126.)

3 Avocado and coconut popsicles
These are fun to make and eat. Why would you think of going back to sugar, right? (See page 158.)

WEEK 8

Hooray!

By the time you get to this page I'm truly hoping sugar is out of your system and that you're alive to sugar and your new (vibrant) body. This, my friends, is wonderful!!

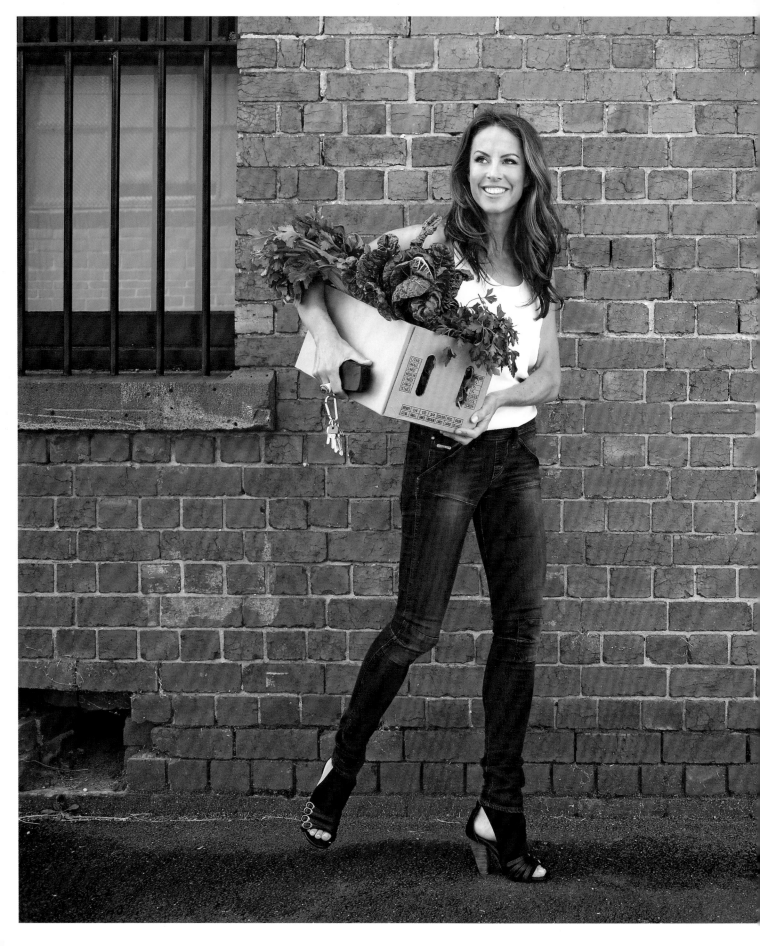

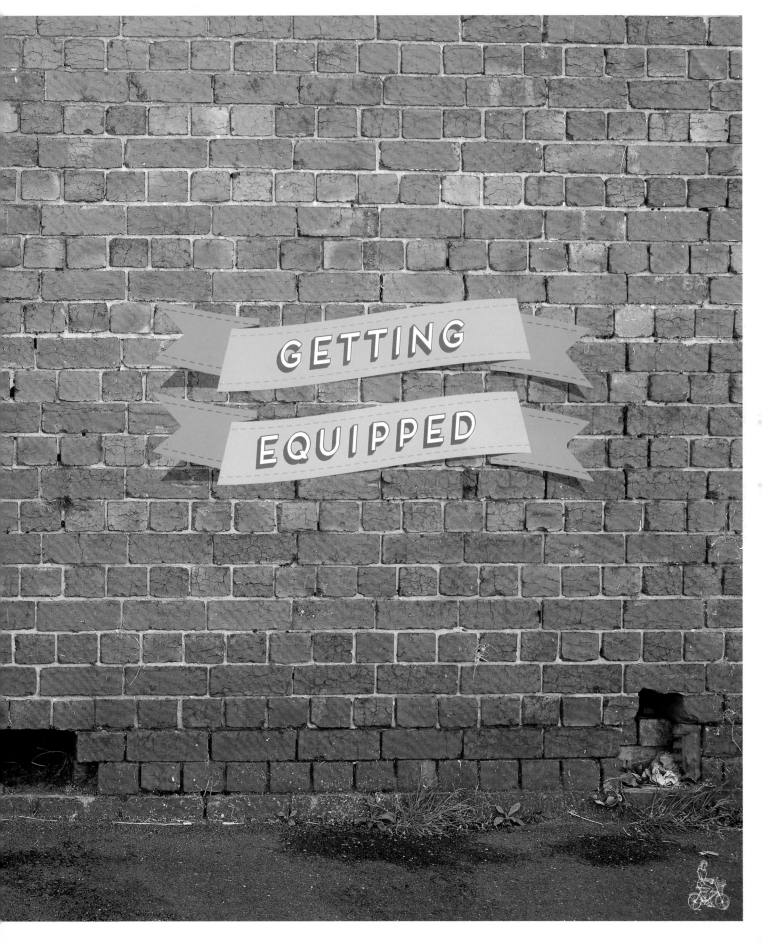

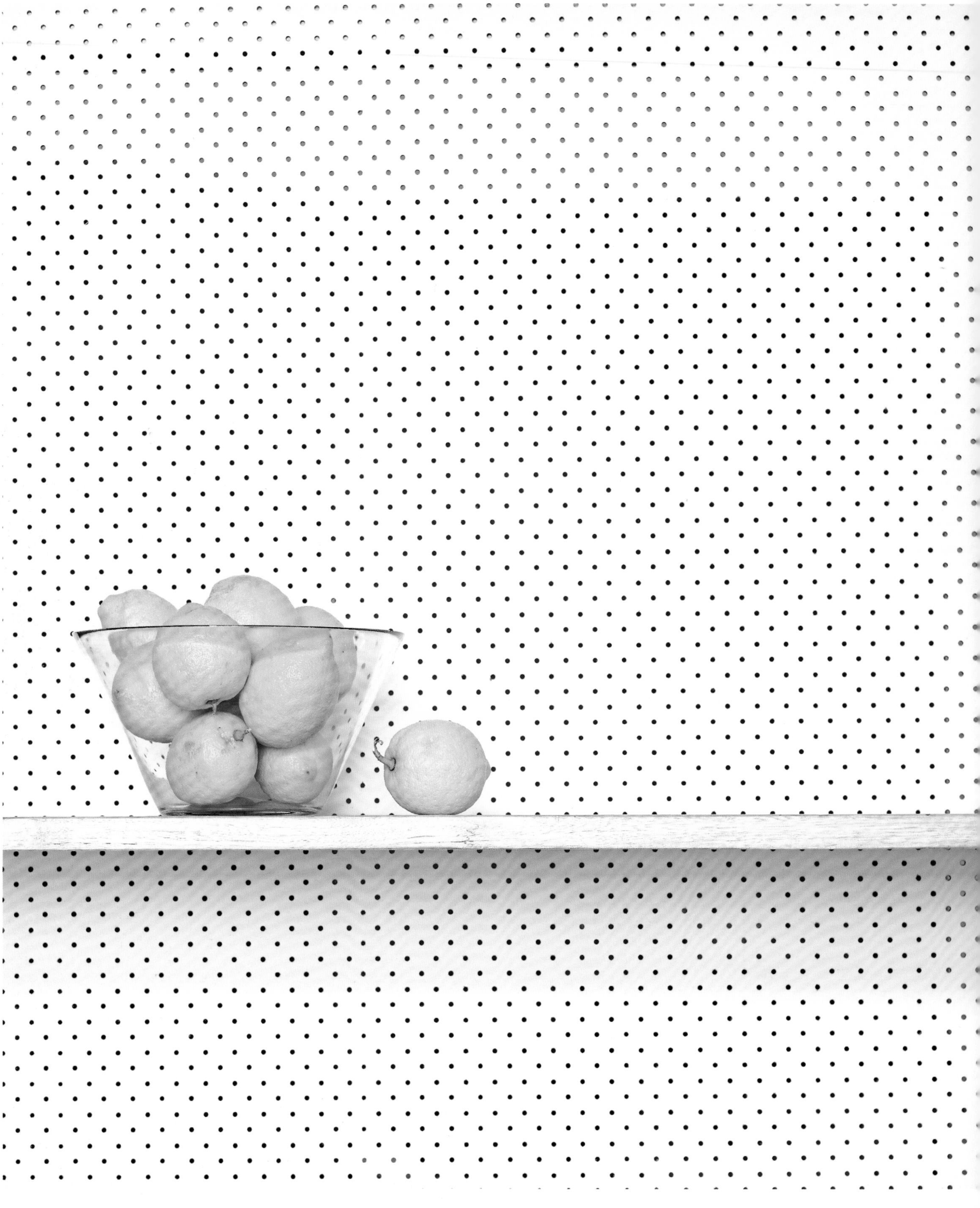

BEFORE WE START, TAKE SOME TIME TO GET PRIMED

A quick two notes:

1. I hate waste...

So I've devised recipes that use the same core ingredients over and over, in different ways. Some might not be familiar to you, or might be a little hard to find in your neighborhood. You might like to buy one or two at a time and see what grabs your fancy. I don't deal in "exacts," so many ingredients in my recipes can actually be replaced if you've run out or don't want to buy a whole box of new stuff.

2. I love efficiency...

So I've devised recipes that use bits and pieces that can be prepared in advance and kept on hand, ready to go.

Just so you know...

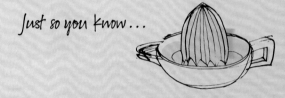

✽ A SIMPLE KITCHEN KIT ✽

This is not a complete list of what you *must* have in your kitchen to successfully cook without sugar. It's more of a heads-up on what I find useful to have on hand for a sugar-free future. I'm not a fan of going overboard with kitchen stash. A bulging cupboard of waffle-makers and grapefruit de-pithers is just depressingly wasteful. There is an elegant joy to be gleaned from using as few dishes as possible, and many of my recipes are designed to be made in one bowl or pan. However, there are some bits and pieces you might like to build up into a kitchen kit.

- Good-quality big knife. (Preferably ceramic—they are impervious to chemical reactions with either acidic or alkaline foods. Your food won't react to the knife, wilt or oxidize.)

- Good-quality small vegetable knife (ceramic).

- Medium-sized saucepan with a double steamer.

- Immersion blender (these are sold individually, or as part of a blender ensemble).

- Small skillet or frying pan (preferably a heavy cast-iron one).

- Medium-sized frying pan (as above), preferably with a lid.

- 9 in. baking dish (square or round; ceramic or glass is best).

- Baking tray/sheet (preferably stainless steel).

- Big soup pot.

- High-powered blender. If you are going to invest in one thing, it should be this. A standard blender is fine, but the high-powered versions can be used to make everything from nut butters to vegetable smoothies, soups and lemon zest. When buying a blender, look out for a style that allows you to put everything into the one vessel and then pour directly from it. You'll thank me for this tip down the road—it saves on cooking steps . . . and washing up!

Your freezer is about to become your new friend. Having a fully stocked freezer will help when using this cookbook, and dozens of the recipes refer back to these staples over and over (so best get stocked in advance!). But also:

▶ A full freezer is a green freezer. Freezers work more efficiently when they're full. Solids freeze at a lower temperature than air does, so it's actually a good thing to stock up your freezer and use it as a storage area.

▶ Freezing saves time and money because it allows you to buy stuff in bulk when it's on sale or in season. I think one of the worst food crimes is to have two heads of broccoli in the crisper that you ignore, and so you leave them another day or two until finally you have to toss them out. Parcook and freeze your veggies as soon as you buy them and you can live your week guilt-free (see opposite page).

▶ Many foods are best when frozen—frozen tofu, for instance, stir-fries better. Nuts are crisper. Also, many starchy vegetables, such as corn and peas, are better frozen than fresh because freezing stops the starch from breaking down into sugars.

TIP

WATCH OUT FOR "FREEZER BURN" (WHERE FOOD BECOMES DISCOLORED AND DEHYDRATED BECAUSE IT IS NOT PROPERLY SEALED IN THE FREEZER). MAKE SURE EVERY-THING IS COVERED, AND FILL CONTAINERS TO THE TOP. STORE SAUCES AND PESTO WITH A LAYER OF OIL ON TOP, AND TOP OFF COOKED BEANS AND RICE WITH A LITTLE WATER, SO THERE IS NO AIR LEFT IN THE CONTAINER.

SQUASH PURÉE

A whole bunch of my recipes use squash that's been blended into a smooth paste—for sublime, low-fructose sweetness. It's handy to have a stash of it, divided into 1-cup batches, in your freezer, ready to go.

1 large butternut or kabocha squash, cut into 4 big wedges

2 tablespoons olive oil

pinch of salt

Preheat the oven to 350°F. Scoop out and discard the squash seeds and strings. Put the squash wedges on a baking tray, then rub with the olive oil and salt. Bake on the middle oven rack until tender—about 1 hour. (If you're pressed for time, cut the squash into smaller chunks and bake for 30 minutes.) Scoop out the flesh and purée using an immersion blender or mash well by hand. Once cool, store in 1-cup batches in the freezer in zip-lock bags or sealed containers.

VARIATION

TO MAKE SWEET POTATO PURÉE, PEEL AND CHOP INTO CHUNKS. EITHER BAKE AND PURÉE AS ABOVE, OR SIMPLY BOIL, DRAIN AND PURÉE.

PARCOOKED-AND-FROZEN VEGETABLES

Many of my recipes call for these handy additions. Again, cook in a big batch and store in the freezer.

Buy a stash of veggies. Stock up on your favorite vegetables when they are in season or on special. Organic veggies can often be really cheap at certain times of the year—invest when they are. Mix it up. Broccoli, spinach, kale, beans and cauliflower work really well as a mixture, but you can try other veggies too.

Blanch them to 60% done. Using a saucepan with a steamer (or double steamer), steam the veggies for 1–2 minutes, then rinse in cold water to stop the cooking process.

Drain and freeze in portions. I divide mine into per-serve portions and put them in zip-lock bags. You can also dump them all into one large container and "break off" what you need as you go, as you would frozen peas.

NOTE

TO PARCOOK FRESH BEETS, SIMPLY PLACE UNPEELED, WHOLE, SCRUBBED BEETS ON A BAKING TRAY (NO OIL, NO SALT, NO BAKING PAPER) AND COOK IN THE OVEN ON 350°F FOR 15 TO 20 MINUTES, UNTIL JUST TENDER. LET COOL AND PEEL (I DON'T, I LIKE THE TEXTURE OF THE SKIN), THEN PLACE IN THE FREEZER.

SPROUTED NUTS AND SEEDS

You can buy sprouted nuts and seeds in health food shops, but they're expensive. It's much cheaper to make your own in bulk. You can make a batch of these and store them in the freezer—they keep fresher for longer and are crunchier! Plus you can eat them straight from the freezer, as they don't actually freeze.

So, what are sprouted nuts? Let me explain. Nuts and seeds contain poisons in the husk that can make them tough to digest. Soaking then drying them causes them to sprout, which activates enzymes that make them easier to digest and metabolize. The more enzymes you get from food, the less your own body's enzymes are required to break down food, and this will keep you younger, longer. Sprouting also produces a crunchier, slightly toasty version of the original nut or seed. Almonds, walnuts, pistachios, pecans and pumpkin seeds work best—the "oily" nuts such as macadamias or cashews can go a little soggy, and must be soaked for no longer than 6 hours.

1 x bag of non-oily nuts or seeds (e.g., almonds, pumpkin seeds, walnuts)

pinch of sea salt

Soak the nuts or seeds overnight in a covered saucepan of water with the salt. Drain, then spread out on a baking tray (no oil, no baking paper) and dry in the oven for 12–24 hours at the lowest temperature possible (less than 150°F for gas ovens, on the pilot light). When cool, store in a sealed container in the freezer.

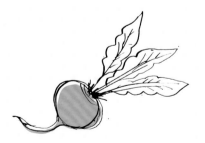

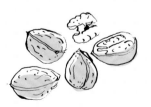

BASIC CHICKEN STOCK

Every freezer should contain stock in 2–3 cup containers, ready to defrost for soups, and in an ice-cube tray, for deglazing and thinning out sauces. Reasons to make your own stock:

▶ Stock is beyond nutritious. It's a condensed cauldron of minerals and electrolytes in a form that is easy for the body to assimilate.

▶ It's great for anyone with digestion issues. Stock has a soothing effect on any areas of inflammation in the gut. That is why it aids digestion and has been known for centuries as a healing remedy for the digestive tract.

▶ The store-bought stuff is full of additives and tastes artificial.

▶ It's economical. You can get about 12 cups of stock and 6–8 portions of meat from one chicken.

▶ Stock is a de-stressor—seriously. It has a natural ingredient that feeds, repairs and calms the mucous lining in the small intestine, which makes up a large part of our nervous system. Ergo all that "chicken soup for the soul" stuff.

▶ It's great for anyone with thyroid or autoimmune issues.

1 whole organic chicken (if you're friendly with your butcher, ask for some extra bony chicken parts: necks, feet, etc.)

1 onion, roughly chopped

2 carrots, roughly chopped

2 celery stalks, chopped

1 teaspoon black peppercorns

3 bay leaves

a few sprigs of thyme (if you have some)

a splash of vinegar

Put all the ingredients in a big soup pot. Cover with 12 to 16 cups of water. The water should cover the ingredients. Bring to a boil, then reduce the heat, cover and simmer for hours—2 is good, 3 is better, about 6 is best. Pull out the chicken and strain the stock, discarding the veggies. Allow to cool, then store in the fridge or freezer. Simple.

Makes about 12 cups

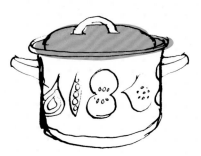

A FEW TIPS FOR MAKING MEAT STOCKS

▶ Adding a little vinegar during cooking draws minerals—particularly calcium, magnesium and potassium—into the broth.

▶ When removing the fat layer, don't get too finicky. Some argue that the fat is the most nutritious stuff.

▶ Always use the whole chicken—especially the bones and joints. Keep the cartilage and joints and eat them after cooking, particularly if you're female. They are the best parts, as they provide the healing substances.

▶ Definitely use an organic, free-range chicken. It's worth the investment. Remember: Everything is going to leach from this thing. Do you really want chemicals and bleaches percolating in your stock?

▶ Stock will keep for about 5 days in the fridge (longer if reboiled) and several months in the freezer.

▶ To thin a savory recipe, toss in a cube of chicken stock from the freezer. In case you're curious, to thin a sweet recipe, toss in a cube of coconut milk from the freezer, or some coconut water.

QUINOA (pronounced KEEN-wah)

What's the big deal with quinoa? Well, it's easy to cook and store in batches in the freezer, but more importantly, if you're gluten-free, it's a great substitute for cereal, oatmeal, couscous and bulgur wheat. If you're grain-free, it can also be suitable as technically it's not a grain (it's a seed) and is easier to digest.

Quinoa is an extremely high-energy food containing all eight amino acids, making it a complete protein, and it has a protein content equal to milk. It's super high in B vitamins, iron, zinc, potassium, calcium and vitamin E. When quinoa is cooked, the outer germ surrounding the seed breaks open to form a crunchy coil while the inner grain becomes soft and translucent, giving it an interesting texture.

VERY IMPORTANT

BEFORE COOKING, QUINOA MUST BE RINSED WELL—PREFERABLY TWICE—TO REMOVE THE TOXIC BUT NATURALLY OCCURRING BITTER COATING CALLED SAPONIN. WHEN YOU RINSE QUINOA, YOU WILL SEE A "SOAPY" SOLUTION IN THE WATER—THAT'S THE SAPONIN.

1 cup quinoa

2 cups water

Rinse the quinoa well. Put it in a saucepan and pour in the water. Cover and bring to a boil, then reduce the heat and simmer, covered, for 15 minutes or until all the water has been absorbed. Remove the pan from the heat and let stand for 5 minutes, covered. Fluff the quinoa with a fork.

Eat immediately or store in the fridge for up to 4 days. (If you prefer, make a larger quantity and freeze in portions.)

Serves 4 (4 cups cooked quinoa)

Because I'm impatient, I sprinkle squash (like this variety of kabocha) with a little salt to speed up the cooking process.

Did I mention I hate waste!? I reserve celery leaves for making stock. I keep them in a zip-lock bag in the freezer, at the ready!

I use my freezer like a pantry, storing pre-cooked stuff as well as grains, seeds and nuts. They last longer, it's a greener way to run my freezer and I have "fresh" staples at the ready. Win! Win! Win!

❋ PANTRY FAVORITES

I abhor the idea of buying an expensive ingredient that I use once and then sits in the cupboard for two years before eventually being tossed. Here is a list of the key ingredients I keep in my pantry or fridge:

▶ **Raw cacao powder and cacao nibs** have a much higher level of antioxidants and minerals than standard cocoa, which has been processed.

▶ **Chia seeds.** These tiny seeds are a super food, being the highest known plant source of omega-3 fatty acids (up to 8 times more than salmon).

TIP

USE CHIA SEEDS TO THICKEN A SOUP, STEW, SMOOTHIES OR CAKE BATTER. THEY CAN ABSORB UP TO 17 TIMES THEIR WEIGHT IN WATER AND WILL SOAK UP A LIQUID IN A MATTER OF MINUTES (ALLOW 2–3 MINUTES FOR THEM TO WORK THEIR MAGIC).

▶ **Nut meals and nut flours** such as almond meal, almond flour and any other kind of nut flour can be used interchangeably. You can also substitute in part quinoa or millet flour or hempseed meal if you run short of a nut flour.

▶ **Nut spreads/butters** include almond, cashew, peanut and macadamia. Only buy versions with no added sugar or salt. Or make your own (see recipe adjacent).

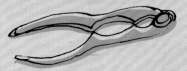

❋ SPREADS AND MILKS

NUT BUTTER

1 bag unsalted nuts (almonds, cashews, macadamias or peanuts—preferably sprouted; see page 59).

Blend in a food processor until the mixture is smooth and creamy. Then store in an airtight container in the fridge for up to three weeks.

CREAM CHEESE

It's so simple to make your own cream cheese. Be sure to use full-fat organic yogurt—I've found that this doesn't work well if you use the commercial stuff.

32 oz. tub full-fat organic plain yogurt

Pour the whole tub of yogurt onto a large handkerchief-sized square of clean cheesecloth or muslin. Bunch the ends like you're tying a sack and secure with an elastic band or string. Suspend the bag over a large bowl—I attach mine to a wooden spoon placed across a bowl, while others hang theirs from a cupboard doorknob, or a chandelier! You're going to be straining out the whey, leaving a beautifully creamy curd in the sack. Drain for 12–24 hours. Store the cream cheese in the fridge for up to 1 month. Keep the whey (you can store it in the freezer) for fermenting vegetables (to make them last longer) or making mayonnaise (see page 67).

THINGS TO DO WITH CREAM CHEESE:

▶ Spread on muffins or toast or pancakes.

▶ Stir in some freshly chopped herbs and salt and sandwich between two seed crackers.

▶ Use to make Endive Sardine Boats (see page 142).

▶ Blend ¼ cup chopped smoked salmon; 1 tablespoon each freshly chopped dill, chives or scallions; a dash of olive oil; and 8 oz. of cream cheese in a food processor. Serve on a rice cake or toast.

ALMOND MILK

Store-bought almond milk can be expensive and often contains added sugar. I always make my own, and it's so quick and simple. You can also do the same with cashews for cashew milk.

3 cups water

1 cup blanched or soaked (overnight) almonds

Boil the water and allow to cool slightly. Blend with the almonds until smooth. Pass the almond milk through a sieve, reserving the pulp. Allow to dry completely and use as almond meal.

Makes about 3½ cups

✳ SPROUTS

I avoid eating too many legumes as I find them rough on my digestive system. Sprouting is certainly the best approach I've found for making them a smoother experience. First, why sprout?

▶ Sprouting kills toxins. Phytic acid—a toxin found in the fiber of legumes—leaches calcium, magnesium, iron, copper and zinc from our bodies. Not great. Sprouting neutralizes this nasty acid (as does soaking before cooking). It also inactivates aflatoxins—potent carcinogens—in grains.

▶ Sprouting increases vitamins. It increases the amount of B vitamins and carotene in the little beady things. Vitamin C is also created in the process.

▶ Sprouting (almost) fixes the flatulence issue because the complex sugars responsible for intestinal gas are broken down into simpler glucose molecules.

▶ Sprouting alkalizes. Legumes tend to be acid-forming but by sprouting them you are effectively making a plant . . . and plants are always alkalizing.

▶ Sprouting increases enzymes. Legumes contain enzyme inhibitors, which unfortunately not only inhibit enzymes in the actual seed but can also inhibit your own valuable enzymes once they have been eaten. So sprouting first neutralizes these while also adding extra enzymes into your system. This helps digestion immeasurably.

▶ Sprouting slows aging. In a nutshell, more enzymes = less aging (a simplistic reading of things, to be sure).

BUT A WORD OF CAUTION ✳

YOU DON'T WANT TO EAT TOO MANY RAW SPROUTED LEGUMES. THEY STILL CONTAIN SOME TOXINS. THE BEST IDEA IS TO ALSO COOK YOUR SPROUTS WHERE POSSIBLE. I BRAISE OR STEAM MINE, OR ADD THEM TO STEWS AND SOUPS. SEE BELOW FOR MORE IDEAS.

SPROUTED LEGUMES

1 cup dried legumes (chickpeas, brown lentils, peas, adzuki beans, and mung beans all work really well)

Soak the legumes in water overnight. In the morning, drain and rinse in a wire sieve. Leaving the legumes in the sieve, prop the sieve over a bowl and put a saucepan lid over the top. Leave on the counter for 2–3 days, rinsing twice a day (I rinse really well, filling the bowl with water over the legumes and stirring up a little before draining). In summer, you'll need to rinse more often. White shoots will start to form after a day or so. Once they're about ¼ in. long, put in a storage container in the fridge for 3–4 days.

THINGS TO DO WITH SPROUTS:

Steam lightly and then sprinkle on a salad.

Toss through stir-fries, casseroles or soups.

For a snack, braise in a little chicken stock (I freeze stock in ice-cube trays for just this purpose) and add a dash of liquid aminos or tamari.

Add to a mish-mash meal. Steam some veggies (broccoli or zucchini) and the sprouts or braise as above, and then toss with ½ chopped avocado, feta, arugula and some capers.

❋ COOKING OILS

There is some conjecture about the best oils to use in cooking. Smoke point (the temperature at which the oil begins to smoke) determines some people's thinking, while stability and fatty-acid-chain composition determine things for others. Here's my advice:

- **Avocado oil** can be used for baking and pouring (i.e., used cold).

- **Butter** is great for baking, cooking (at low–medium temperatures only) and greasing trays and pans.

- **Coconut oil** is the best oil for greasing trays and pans, and can also be used for baking and cooking.

- **Ghee** can be used for cooking and for greasing trays and pans.

- **Macadamia oil** is good for baking, cooking and pouring (i.e., used cold).

- **Olive oil** is used for cooking (at low–medium temperatures only), greasing trays and pans and pouring (i.e., used cold).

Never touch seed oils such as canola, sunflower and soy. (See page 22 for more info.)

TIP

TRY PUTTING A DAB OF COCONUT OIL IN YOUR CAKE OR MUFFIN TIN, THEN POPPING THE TIN IN THE OVEN AS IT'S PREHEATING, TO MELT THE OIL. REMOVE AFTER A MINUTE AND SWIRL. VOILÀ! PAN GREASED.

NOTE

AVOCADO OIL, BUTTER, COCONUT OIL AND MACADAMIA OIL ARE GENERALLY USED FOR BAKING AS THEY HAVE HIGH HEAT POINTS AND CAN BE USED INTERCHANGEABLY. JUST BEAR IN MIND THAT COCONUT AND MACADAMIA OILS AREN'T A NEUTRAL FLAVOR—BUT THIS CAN WORK IN YOUR FAVOR IF YOU'RE BAKING A SWEET RECIPE.

❋ SWEETENERS

Here are some simple conversions to help you cook with sweeteners.

STEVIA

When I refer to stevia in this book, I mean the granulated form unless specified otherwise. Most stevia granules you can use as you would sugar, although I tend to use a little less because that's my taste preference these days. If you're using the liquid form, keep in mind these conversions:

1 cup sugar/granulated stevia = 1 teaspoon liquid stevia

1 tablespoon sugar/granulated stevia = 6–9 drops liquid stevia

1 teaspoon sugar/granulated stevia = 2–4 drops liquid stevia

BROWN RICE SYRUP

Use this in place of sugar or honey in recipes, roughly in a 1:1 ratio. Some people say brown rice syrup is less sweet than honey or sugar, but I beg to differ, and I tend to put less of it in my recipes than many others would. Perhaps it's because my tastebuds have shifted!

GLUCOSE SYRUP OR DEXTROSE

David Gillespie, author of *Sweet Poison* and *Big Fat Lies*, is a big fan of using dextrose, which is generally called "glucose syrup," for baking. You can find it in some supermarkets in the baking section, at some baking supply and craft stores, or online. (See Resources, page 205). I personally don't cook with it (see page 43), but I know some folks are fans. So here are some tips for converting recipes yourself:

Replace sugar for dextrose 1:1.

Increase the wet ingredients and use an extra egg.

Don't overbeat once flour has been added.

Watch it doesn't burn.

Don't store for too long, and store in the fridge. Sugar is a preservative, but dextrose isn't.

For more information on sugar alternatives, see page 43.

Again, just start with some good staples:

▸ **The grounds**—cinnamon, cumin, nutmeg, allspice, ginger, chili, paprika, salt and pepper.

▸ **The blends**—five-spice mix, ras el hanout, garam masala and za'atar. (I like to have two spice blends in my cupboard at a time. I go through phases, and play with one blend on popcorn, veggie chips, soups and more, then move on to the other when I've almost run out.)

▸ **Dulse flakes**—dried red seaweed, great for sprinkling on soups, popcorn and other savory snacks. High in vitamins, minerals and protein.

▸ **Salt**—it's always best to use pure rock salt or sea salt (processed table salt lacks many of the minerals found in rock and sea salt).

▸ **Vanilla powder**—made from ground vanilla beans. I tend to use this rather than vanilla extract, which often contains added sugar. The powder can be hard to find, so scour the health food shops and keep it safe and dry.

Packaged sauces are a sugar-quitter's stealth enemy. They are full of sugar, wrapped up in a seductive, savory and often "low-fat" packaging. My advice is to avoid all commercial sauces apart from these:

▸ **Mustard**—whole grain, French, Dijon . . . Play with different options and make simple dressings by blending mustard, olive oil, lemon juice and crushed garlic and shaking in a jar.

▸ **Apple cider vinegar**—great for salad dressings, marinades and chutneys.

▸ **Tamari**—a wheat-free, sugar-free version of soy sauce.

FOUR SAUCES TO TRY

HOMEMADE MAYONNAISE

This recipe lists whey as an optional ingredient. Mayonnaise made with whey will keep for 2–3 months longer than mayonnaise made without, which normally only lasts 2–3 weeks. You can use the whey that is left over from making your own cream cheese (see page 64). If you don't have any whey, that's fine, but use up the mayonnaise within a week or two.

1 egg

1 teaspoon Dijon mustard

1 tablespoon lemon juice

1 tablespoon whey (optional)

pinch of salt

1 cup extra-virgin olive oil

Blend all the ingredients except the oil for 30 seconds in a food processer on low speed. With the motor running, add the oil in a slow drizzle until the mayo is thick and smooth. If you included the whey, cover the mayonnaise and allow to sit on your counter for 7 hours before refrigerating—this activates the enzymes in the whey.

Makes about 1⅓ cups

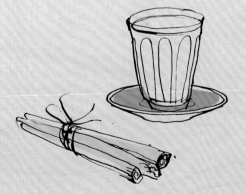

HOMEMADE KETCHUP

2 cans tomatoes or 28 ounces tomato puree or crushed tomatoes

½ onion, chopped

⅓ cup apple cider vinegar

1 tablespoon brown rice syrup (or 2 teaspoons granulated stevia)

1 teaspoon ground allspice

1 teaspoon ground cinnamon

1 teaspoon ground cloves

1 teaspoon cayenne pepper

salt and freshly ground black pepper, to taste

Bring all the ingredients to a boil in a saucepan, stirring to dissolve the spices. Reduce the heat and simmer for about 50 minutes, until the sauce reduces by almost half and is quite thick. Blend with an immersion blender or in a food processer. If the ketchup is still a bit runny, return it to the heat for a little longer. Store in a clean glass jar in the fridge for up to 1 month. (I divide my mixture and freeze half so it doesn't spoil.)

Makes about 2 cups

NOTE

YOU CAN ALSO DO THIS IN A SLOW COOKER: COOK ALL THE INGREDIENTS ON HIGH FOR 2–2½ HOURS. AFTER BLENDING, YOU MIGHT WANT TO RETURN IT TO THE COOKER FOR ANOTHER 30 MINUTES, WITHOUT THE LID, TO THICKEN IT.

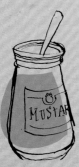

HOMEMADE BARBEQUE SAUCE

1 cup homemade ketchup (see left)

2 tablespoons apple cider vinegar

1 teaspoon tabasco sauce

1 clove garlic, minced

1 tablespoon paprika

2 tablespoons chili powder

Mix all the ingredients and store in a clean glass jar in the fridge for up to 1 month.

Makes about 1⅓ cups

BERRY GROWN-UP SAUCE

Great as a sweet coulis accompaniment to desserts or spooned over yogurt.

2 cups frozen berries

1 tablespoon brown rice syrup

1 teaspoon finely grated fresh ginger

½ teaspoon grated orange zest

1 star anise, finely crushed

¼ teaspoon ground cinnamon

Combine all the ingredients in a small saucepan and bring to a boil. Lower the heat and simmer for 5–10 minutes. Serve warm or cool. Store in a clean glass jar in the fridge for up to 2 weeks.

Makes about 2 cups

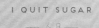

▶ **Coconut flour.** There are three things you should know before using coconut flour: it's sweet (so it's great for baking); it soaks up a lot of liquid, which means you may have to add extra liquid—such as an egg or some coconut water—if the mixture starts to cake; and it produces chewy rather than fluffy baked goods. Arrowroot or tapioca can be substituted for coconut flour—they are all thickening agents.

▶ **Unsweetened shredded or desiccated coconut.** Great for baking.

▶ **Unsweetened coconut flakes.** These aren't the same as unsweetened desiccated or shredded coconut—they're chunkier "scrapings."

▶ **Coconut cream.** Thicker than coconut milk, this is perfect for creamy curry sauces, and for using instead of cream.

▶ **Coconut water.** Great on its own or can be used as a substitute for milk.

These nutrient-rich powders can be a quick and easy way to supplement your diet with the necessary vitamins, minerals, proteins and other essentials that your body needs, especially during the detox period in week 5. But they are supplements, not food substitutes, so it's important to still eat a healthy, balanced diet. Most are available at health food stores and some pharmacies. (See also Resources, page 205.) These are the ones I regularly use:

▶ **Green powders**—a concentrated blend of a variety of green vegetables and plants.

▶ **Spirulina powder**—a highly nutritious saltwater micro plant.

▶ **Protein powder**—helps stimulate metabolism of fat and boosts immune system.

▶ **Maca powder**—a plant-based super food from South America.

▶ **Acai powder**—a berry super food from the Amazon, rich in antioxidants.

▶ **Slippery elm powder**—made from the bark of the slippery elm tree; as well as rich in nutrients, it is also high in fiber and aids digestion.

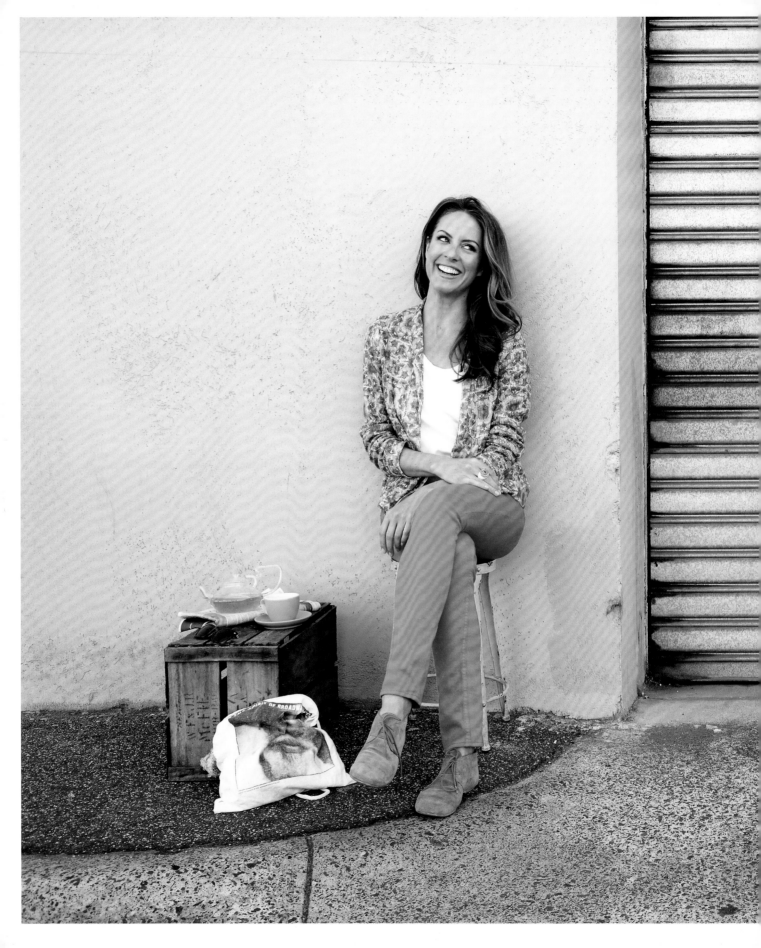

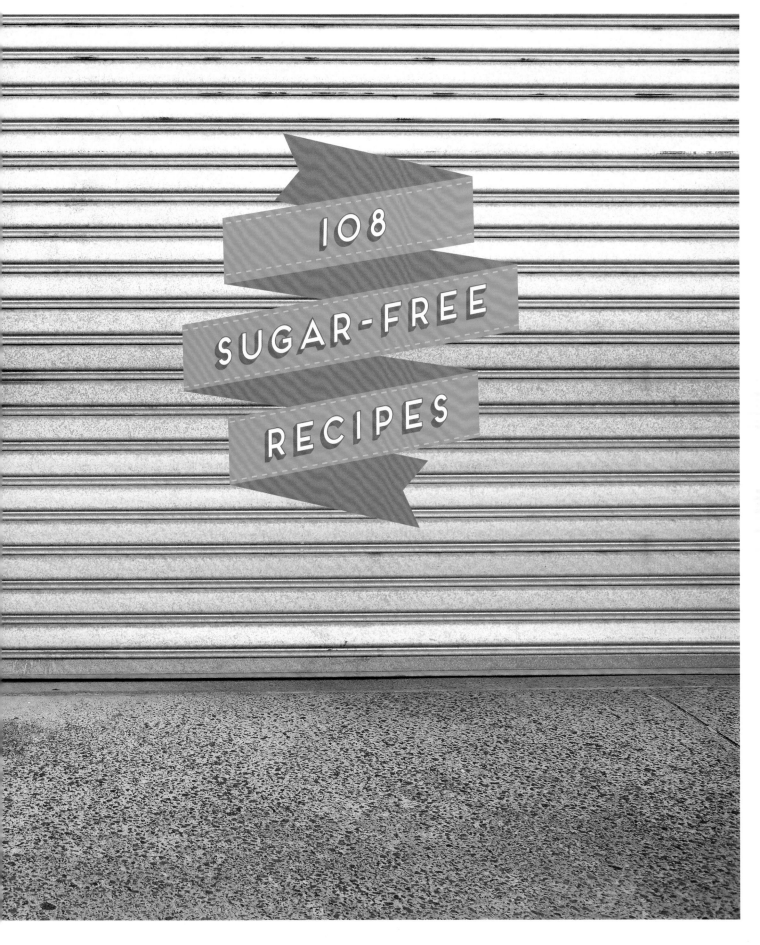

108
SUGAR-FREE
RECIPES

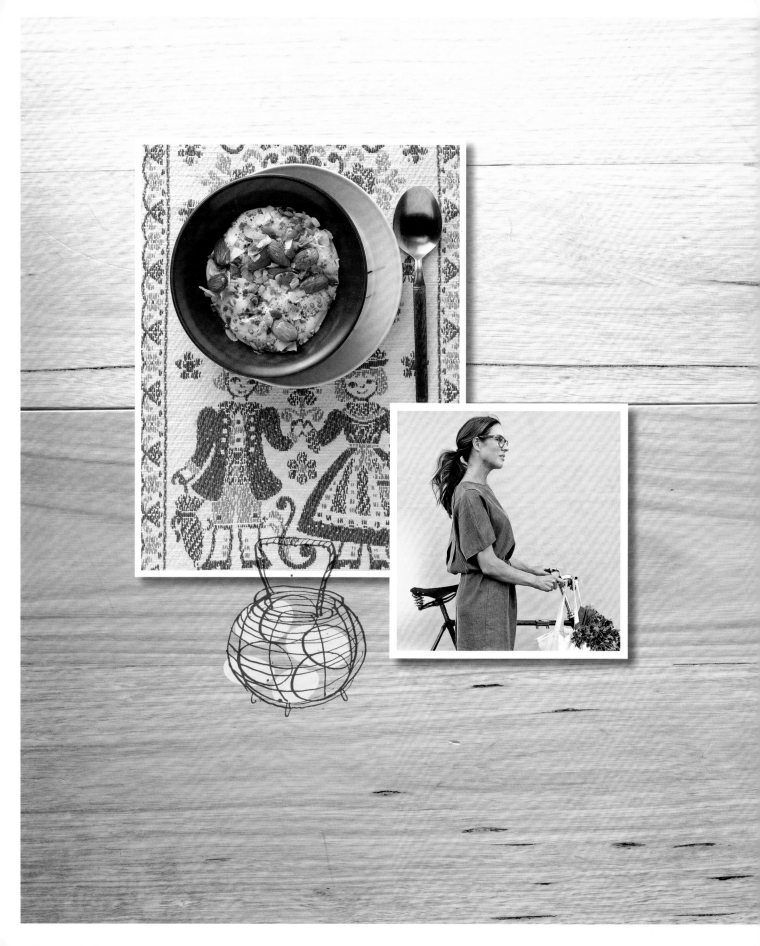

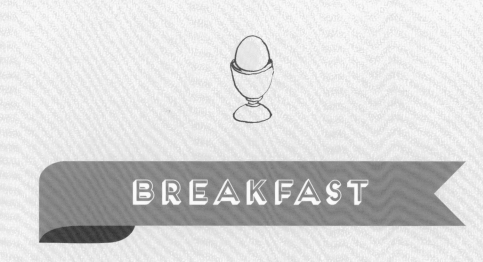

BREAKFAST

The biggest dilemma for anyone quitting sugar is what you are going to eat for breakfast. If you can't have fruit, juice, raisin toast, granola, cereal, muffins, banana bread or pancakes, what's left?

Well, a lot, actually. It means letting go of the notion of sugar- and starch-based "breakfast foods"—a concept invented by breakfast cereal companies in the 1940s. Seriously.

The aim at breakfast time is to eat plenty of protein and good fats. Eating these slow-burning fuels is like throwing a sturdy log onto your metabolic fire that will keep you fueled until lunch (sugars and starches are the equivalent of paper and twigs). I no longer hold on to the idea that my first meal of the day should be shaken from a box. Since quitting sugar, my breakfast is now all about eggs, cheese, yogurt, bacon, coconut and nuts, along with a lot of vegetables and a little low-sugar fruit, such as berries or kiwifruit.

Am I happier? Oh, yes.

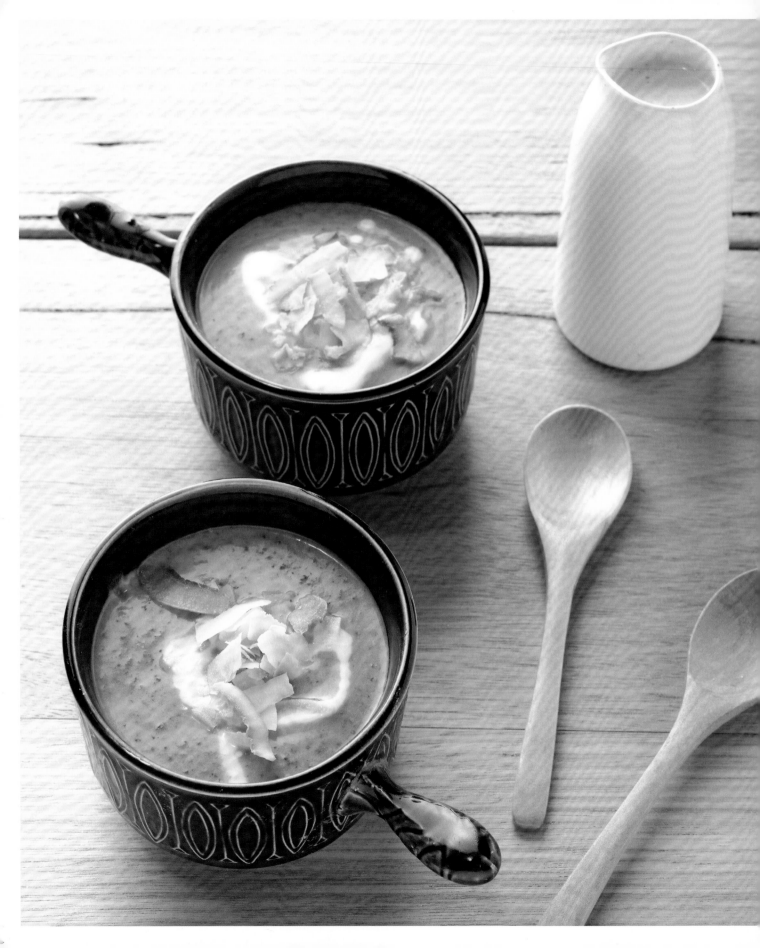

PUMPKIN PIE "OATMEAL"

Have you ever checked out lush foodie blog My New Roots? If not, you should. Creator Sarah Britton's deep understanding of comforting foods sings from the pages. This is one of her personal favorites, which I have adjusted to make the recipe fructose-free. It really is like a pumpkin pie in a bowl!

INGREDIENTS

½ cup amaranth, soaked for 8–24 hours (the longer, the better)

1 cup coconut milk, plus extra for serving

⅓ cup canned unsweetened pumpkin purée or Squash Purée (see page 58)

pinch of salt

pinch of ground cinnamon

pinch of ground nutmeg

pinch of ground ginger

pinch of ground allspice

pinch of vanilla powder

½ teaspoon granulated stevia (optional)

⅓ cup unsweetened coconut flakes, toasted

SERVES 2

METHOD

Drain and rinse the amaranth. Combine in a saucepan with the coconut milk, pumpkin purée, salt, spices and vanilla powder. Bring to a boil, then cover and simmer on the lowest heat for 15 minutes, stirring often to prevent scorching. Watch to see if the liquid level becomes too low; if it does, add a little extra coconut milk or water. Turn off the heat and let sit for 10 minutes with the lid on to thicken. Sweeten with the stevia if desired, then serve drizzled with coconut milk and sprinkled with the coconut flakes.

VARIATION
If you don't have amaranth (a gluten-free grain), you could substitute 1 cup oats.

COCO-NUTTY GRANOLA

The brown rice syrup in this recipe is optional—I personally don't sweeten my granola at all. Perhaps make half a batch with the syrup, half without, and see what you like. I like to eat this granola with yogurt—nice and chunky.

INGREDIENTS

3 cups unsweetened coconut flakes
2 cups almonds, cashews, pecans, walnuts, pumpkin seeds (preferably sprouted; see page 59), roughly chopped (you can use either one type or a mixture)
2 tablespoons chia seeds
1 teaspoon ground cinnamon (optional)
5–7 tablespoons coconut oil or butter, melted
3 tablespoons brown rice syrup (optional)

MAKES 5 CUPS

METHOD

Preheat the oven to 250°F and line a baking tray with baking paper. Combine all the ingredients, then spread evenly on the tray. Bake for 15–20 minutes, until golden, turning halfway through the cooking time. I like to bake mine until quite dark—the darker it is, the crunchier. Remove from the oven and allow to cool, then eat while it's still crispy.

VARIATIONS

If you wish to add rolled oats, toss 2 cups into the bowl with the rest of the ingredients, and add a little more oil and syrup.

To make chocolate granola clusters, mix in ½ cup raw cacao powder and 2 tablespoons cacao nibs with the rest of the ingredients before baking. Place the clusters on top of coconut yogurt as a dessert!

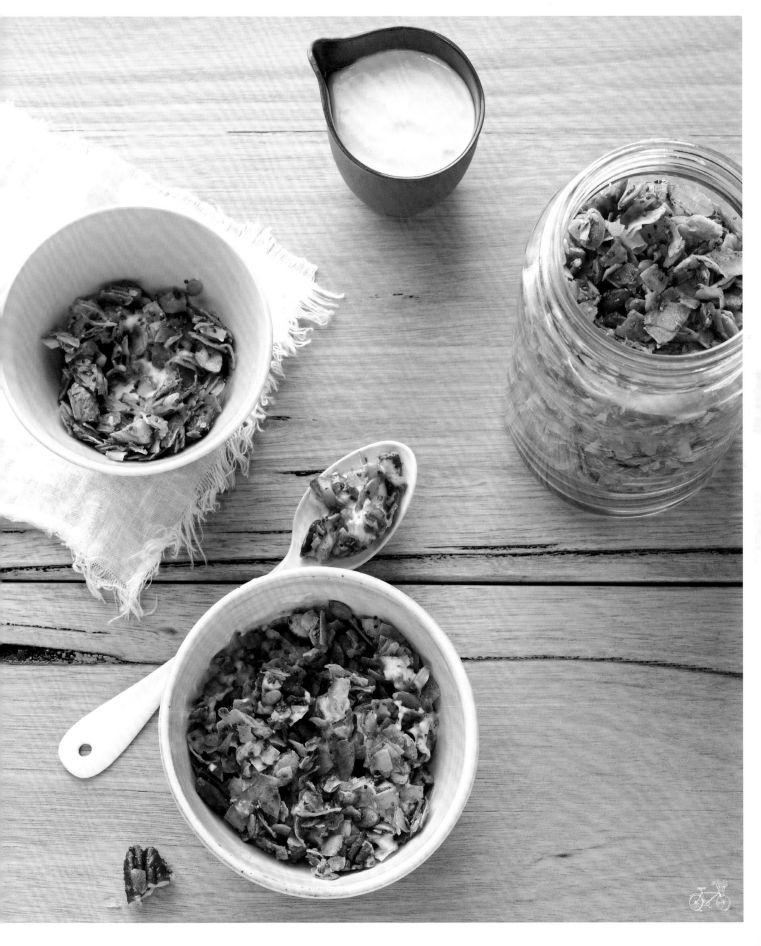

SIMPLE BREAKFAST IDEAS

⇨ BREAKFAST IS THE HARDEST MEAL OF THE DAY TO ADJUST TO
WHEN QUITTING SUGAR BECAUSE MOST "BREAKFAST FOODS"
ARE LADEN WITH SUGAR (A LOT OF IT HIDDEN). ⇦

Some "healthy" granolas (even the American Heart Association–approved ones) contain more sugar than Coco Puffs! And as we know, fruit juices can contain more sugar than soda. You have to be careful with this first meal of the day.

No one has ever said you have to have cereal or fruit for breakfast, so get imaginative. The trick is to include healthy fats and protein in each meal. Here are some simple ideas you can play with to get started.

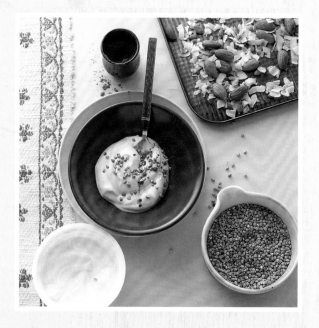

AT HOME

- Millet toast with cashew or almond butter, or tahini.
- Avocado and pumpkin seeds on toast.
- Avocado and cheese melt (I love the way avocado goes soft and gooey when heated).
- Oatmeal "sweetened" with a little coconut milk and cinnamon, or with yogurt and nuts.
- Buckwheat groats (see Resources, page 205), unsweetened coconut (flakes, shredded or desiccated) and pumpkin seeds (or whatever nuts or seeds you have in the cupboard) toasted in a non-stick pan, then sprinkled over yogurt and mashed with either cinnamon or raw cacao powder and/or a drizzle of macadamia oil (pictured at left).
- Cream cheese or coconut cream and frozen berries mashed in a cup.
- In a hot pan, heat leftover veggies with an egg tossed through (who says you can't do veggies for breakfast?).

- A big chunk of feta with some chopped tomato, sardines and olives, with olive oil and salt over the top, Greek style.
- A smoothie (coconut- or yogurt-based). See pages 109–18 for recipe ideas.
- Sugar-free (and fruit-free) granola. There is a range on the market these days. Or try my granola (see page 76).
- Endive Sardine Boats (see page 142). I eat these for breakfast on a weekly basis!
- Pea, Herb and Almond Crush (see page 141), spread on toast.
- Cheesy Biscuits (see page 153). An amazing breakfast food. Eat straight from the oven and serve with some fresh tomato.

EATING OUT

- Eggs and bacon on toast, with healthy extras such as mushrooms, spinach and avocado.
- Smoked salmon on toast.
- Ham and cheese toastie.
- Vegetable juice (but be warned: carrot and beet are almost as high in sugar as fruit is).
- Oatmeal with berries and yogurt, but only if both the berries and yogurt are unsweetened. (It's hard to find—and justify paying for—café oatmeal that isn't super-sweetened with banana and honey and so on. I tend to avoid it.)

- A glass of milk. With some cinnamon. You'd be surprised how good this is. And what café doesn't have milk?
- If you don't eat bread (I personally can't), take your own gluten-free bread (I wrap two slices in foil and hand over to the kitchen to be toasted), or ask for your eggs to be served on a bed of spinach instead.

NOTE

BEWARE OF "NO ADDED SUGAR" MUFFINS AND GRANOLAS. THEY ARE RARELY, IF EVER, SUGAR-FREE.

ON THE RUN

- Plain yogurt.
- Nuts (preferably sprouted; see page 59).
- Coconut water.
- A smoothie (see pages 109–18). Add extra chia seeds and ice, then parfreeze in a travel cup or jar with a lid so that it's nice and firm. I do this for plane trips and long drives.
- The Eggy Muggin (page 92) and Cashewy Chia Puddings (page 80) were designed by me for eating on the run!

CASHEWY CHIA PUDDINGS

INGREDIENTS

½ cup chia seeds
1⅔ cups cashew milk (or homemade Almond Milk,
see page 65, or regular milk)
¼ cup frozen berries (optional)
½ teaspoon vanilla powder
granulated stevia, to taste
pinch of salt

SERVES 2

METHOD

Combine all the ingredients in a bowl. Divide between 2 serving bowls and chill before eating.

NOTE

Make the night before to take to work. But add a little more liquid—chia seeds soak up everything in sight. The puddings will keep for a few days in the fridge.

CHEWY SQUASH AND COCONUT MUFFINS

INGREDIENTS

coconut oil or butter for greasing
½ cup butternut or kabocha squash
½ cup coconut flour, sifted
½ cup almond meal, hempseed meal or other nut meal
2 tablespoons granulated stevia
½ cup basil leaves
½ teaspoon baking powder
pinch of vanilla powder
1 teaspoon ground cinnamon
¼ teaspoon ground nutmeg
6 eggs
½ cup plus 2 tablespoons coconut oil, melted
¾ cup walnuts, roughly chopped
splash of coconut water (add more if needed)

❋ **BATCH & FREEZE** | **MAKES** 15

METHOD

Preheat the oven to 375°F and lightly grease 15 muffin cups (or use cupcake papers). Grate the squash (preferably with a food processor). Add the flour, almond meal, stevia, basil, baking powder, vanilla powder and spices to the squash. Whisk the eggs in a separate bowl, then use a wooden spoon to stir the eggs and coconut oil into the squash mixture until the lumps are gone. Gently stir in the walnuts. Add the coconut water, stirring, until the batter is thick. Spoon into the muffin cups and bake for 15–20 minutes. Serve warm or cold.

Remember: Coconut flour produces a chewy muffin (see page 69).

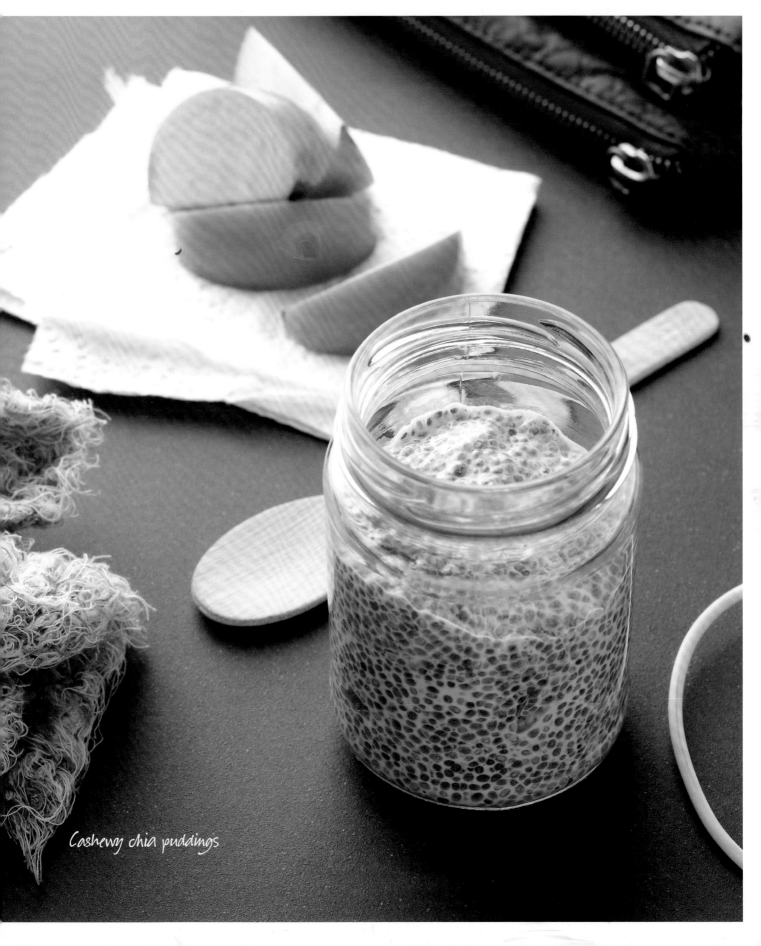

Cashewy chia puddings

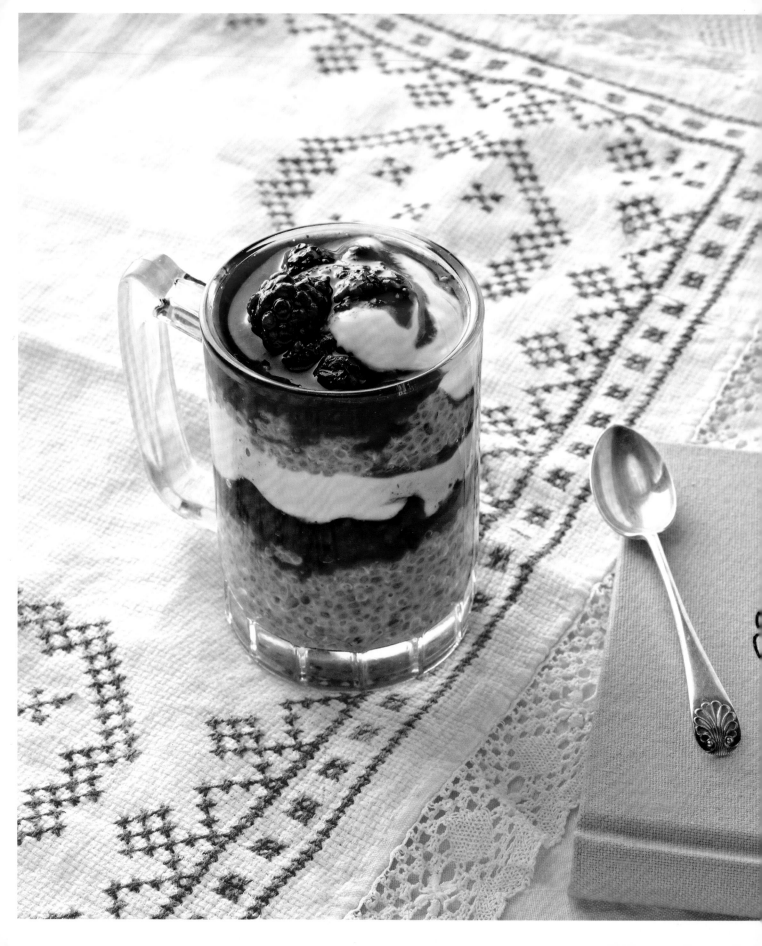

CHIA AND QUINOA PARFAIT

I saw this done with granola in a restaurant in Spain, and decided to do my own sugar-free, densely nutritious version. You need to make these a couple of hours in advance.

INGREDIENTS

½ cup cooked quinoa (see page 61)

3 tablespoons chia seeds

1 tablespoon flaxseeds (linseeds)

1⅔ cups milk or homemade Almond Milk (see page 65) or coconut milk

2 teaspoons raw cacao powder

½ cup full-fat unsweetened thick Greek-style yogurt

½ cup Berry Grown-Up Sauce (see page 68) or 1 handful frozen berries, chopped

SERVES 2

METHOD

Mix the quinoa, chia seeds, flaxseeds, milk and cacao powder well, then put in the fridge for 1–2 hours. To serve, layer with the yogurt and berries in a pretty glass. Get decorative!

POACHED EGGS

Everyone needs to know how to poach an egg, and it's a simple technique. These little parcels of goodness are designed to plop on top of a meal that is otherwise a little lackluster or lacking in protein. You can cook a few at a time and store them in a bowl of cold water in the fridge, where they'll keep for several days.

INGREDIENTS

white vinegar or rice vinegar (optional)

eggs

1–2 EGGS PER PERSON

METHOD

Fill a small shallow frying pan that has a lid with water (or pour water into a wide saucepan to a depth of 2 in.). Bring to a boil. Add a dash of white or rice vinegar if you like—this will help the egg whites to congeal neatly rather than spray out in the pan. Break an egg into a teacup, then tip the egg from the cup into the water. (You can poach a few eggs at a time, if you like.) Turn off the heat immediately and cover the pan tightly. Leave for 3–4 minutes, then remove each egg with a slotted spoon.

TO SERVE, TRY THESE EGGY BREAKFAST BOMBS:

- After removing the eggs from the hot water, use the same pot to steam some frozen peas and chopped zucchini (place a steamer attachment on top). Mix the steamed veggies with a can of tuna, some finely chopped scallions or red onion, and capers. Plop a poached egg on top to serve.

- While the eggs are poaching, sauté some garlic and Swiss chard. Toss in some Parmesan, then plop a poached egg on top to serve.

- I like this idea: poach the egg in a sauce instead of water. I also like the idea of using leftover soup instead of water. Simply heat the soup in a small pan and poach the eggs as above. Serve with a sprinkle of Parmesan.

⇨ *Some of my favorites, clockwise from the top: eggs in soup, peas and spinach with an egg on top, a poached egg on toast.*

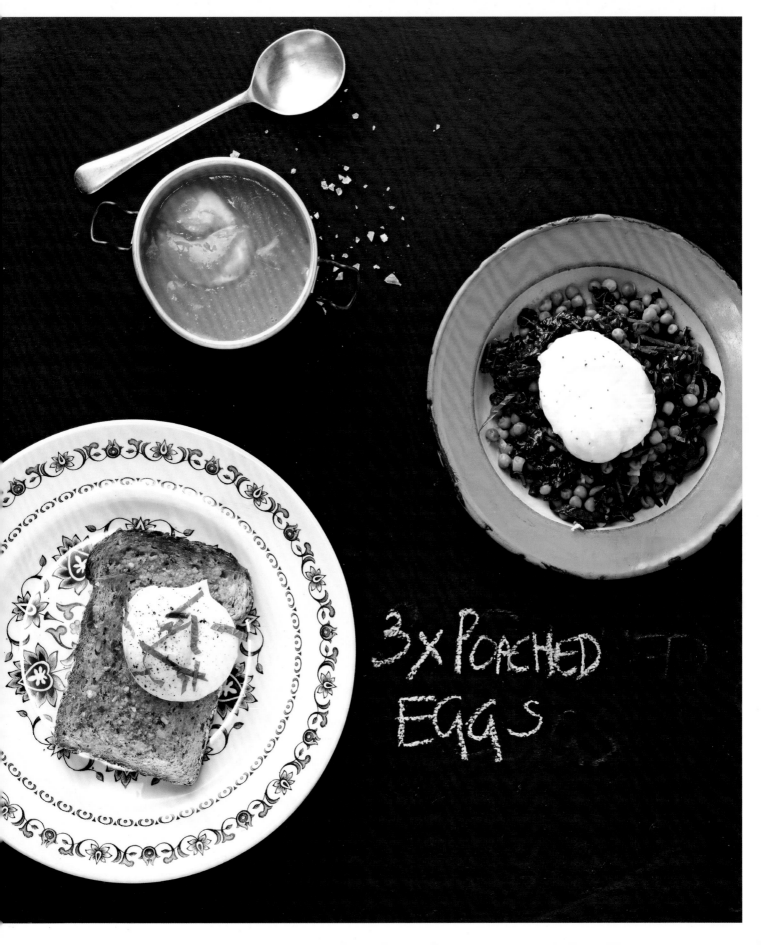

3 x POACHED EGGS

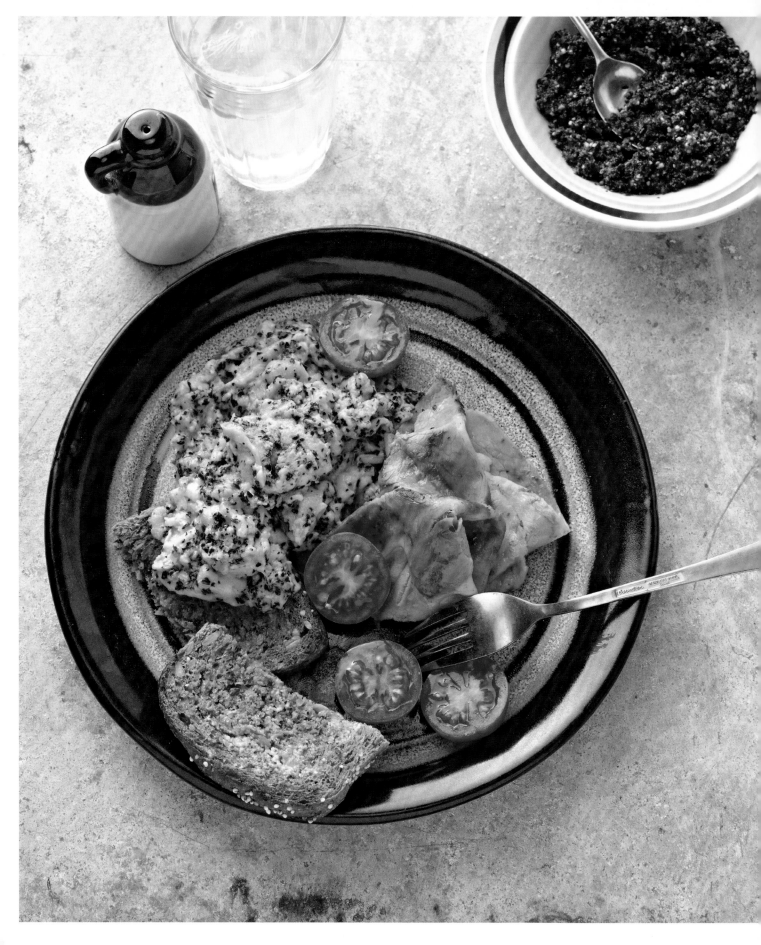

GREEN EGGS WITH HAM

INGREDIENTS

4 eggs

pinch of salt

splash of milk or cream

knob of butter

3 tablespoons Kale Pesto (see page 126)

toast, halved cherry tomatoes and
slices of grilled ham, to serve

SERVES 2

METHOD

Use a fork to lightly mix the eggs, salt and milk or cream in a small bowl—not too much as you want to see a bit of yolk streaked through. Melt the butter in a frying pan over medium heat, then pour in the egg mixture. Once the eggs "take" a little, gently fold and lift using a flat wooden spatula—don't stir. Pause, then fold again. After a minute, add the pesto and fold a little more until the egg mixture is just soft and still a bit runny (about another minute). Remove from the heat and let sit, then gently stir to ensure it is cooked through. Serve with toast, cherry tomato halves and a few slices of grilled ham.

BACON AND EGG "CUPCAKES"

INGREDIENTS

coconut oil or butter for greasing

6 strips bacon

6 eggs

crumbled feta (optional)

chopped chives or other herbs (optional)

MAKES 6

METHOD

Preheat the oven to 400°F and lightly grease a 6-cup muffin pan. Use a bacon strip to line each muffin cup, looping or pressing the bacon around the sides and using any small broken bits to line the bottom. It needn't be a perfect job—feel free to use extra bits to fill in the gaps. If you like your bacon crispy, place the tray in the oven for 5 minutes before continuing. Gently crack 1 egg into each bacon cup, then sprinkle with cheese and herbs if desired. Bake for 15 minutes, until the egg whites are set. Let sit for a minute and then, using a knife or spoon, gently remove the "cupcakes" from the pan. Serve hot or warm.

VARIATION

For a "greener" option, place a small parcooked-and-frozen broccoli floret (see page 59) in each cup. Use only 5 eggs and beat them lightly with a fork before dividing among the 6 cups.

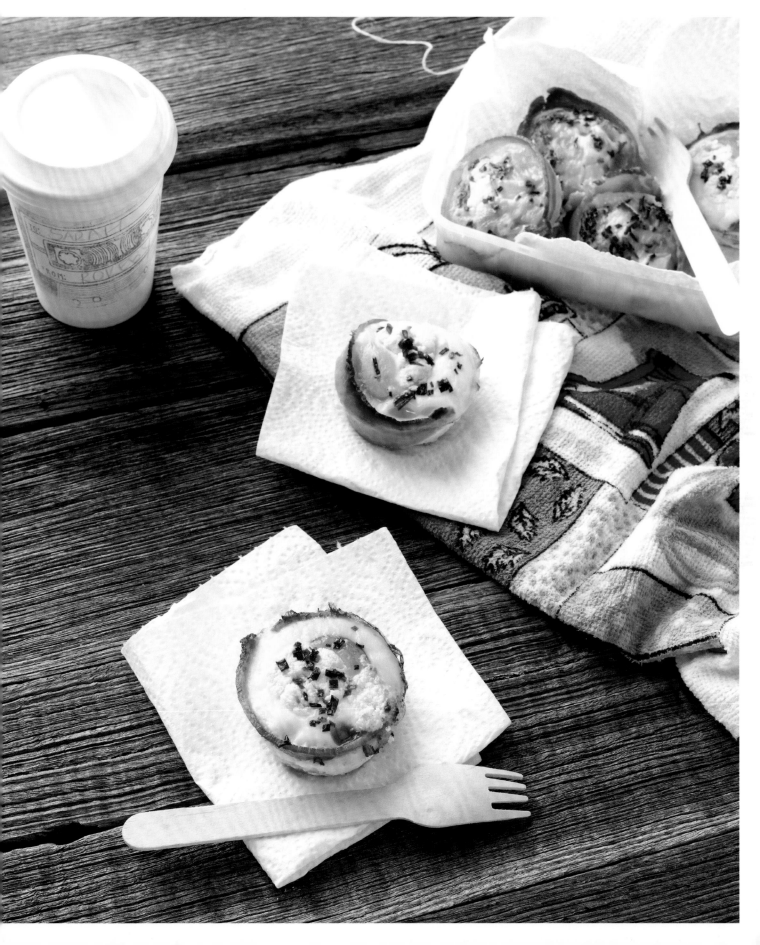

FRITTATINIS

Frittatinis? Yep, mini frittatas!

INGREDIENTS

coconut oil or butter for greasing

8 eggs

2 cups roughly chopped raw vegetables (asparagus, mushrooms, onion, squash, zucchini—whatever you have in the fridge)

6 slices ham or 4 strips bacon, diced

3 scallions, green parts only, sliced, or a handful of basil leaves, chopped

freshly ground black pepper and/or red pepper flakes, to taste

❄ **BATCH & FREEZE** | **MAKES** 12–16

METHOD

Preheat the oven to 325°F and grease a 12-cup muffin pan. Beat the eggs in a large bowl. Finely chop the veggies using a food processor. Add the veggie mix and ham to the eggs, then stir in the scallions, black pepper and/or red pepper flakes and spoon the mixture into the muffin cups. Bake for 12–15 minutes. Eat while warm.

VARIATION

Instead of raw vegetables, use 2 cups chopped leftover or parcooked-and-frozen veggies (see page 59), such as butternut or kabocha squash, sweet potato and broccoli, and toss in a few frozen peas as well. Skip the food processer step.

EASY-PEASY ZUCCHINI BLINIS

INGREDIENTS

2–3 large zucchini
1 tablespoon coconut flour
3 eggs
salt and freshly ground black pepper
coconut oil or butter for frying
homemade Cream Cheese (see page 64)
and chopped chives, to serve

MAKES 8–10

METHOD

Grate the zucchini using a food processor with a shredding disk—you need 2 cups grated zucchini. Sift the coconut flour into the eggs and beat them together until smooth. Mix in the zucchini, salt and pepper. Heat a little oil in a frying pan and spoon in dollops of the batter. Cook until golden on both sides. Serve warm with cream cheese and chives on top.

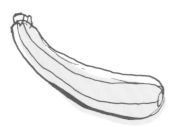

EGGY MUGGIN

Muggins are a muffin-type creation made in a mug—perfect for taking to work or on road trips. Eating while driving isn't great, nor is using a microwave, but if it's the difference between eating a solid breakfast and not. . .

INGREDIENTS

½ cup parcooked-and-frozen veggies (see page 59) (broccoli or Swiss chard works best) or 1 cup fresh baby spinach leaves

small handful of frozen peas

1 egg

pinch of grated Cheddar, Parmesan or feta

MAKES 1

METHOD

Place the vegetables in a large coffee mug with a dash of water. Microwave on high for 30 seconds–1 minute. Crack in the egg, add the cheese and stir loosely. Microwave again for 30 seconds–1 minute; the egg should be fluffy and cooked through. Eat while still warm.

ENERGY MEFFINS

Meffins? Yep, meat muffins!

INGREDIENTS

coconut oil or butter for greasing

1 pound ground pork or beef

1 cup chopped leftover or parcooked-and-frozen veggies (see page 59), such as carrot, squash, peas and zucchini

12 eggs

8 ounces cottage cheese

several tablespoons freshly chopped herbs (I use sage and thyme) and/or 2 teaspoons dried herbs and spices (I like a bit of nutmeg)

handful of grated Cheddar cheese

❄ **BATCH & FREEZE** | **MAKES** 12

METHOD

Preheat the oven to 350°F and lightly grease a 12-cup muffin pan. Brown the meat in a frying pan with a little oil, then remove and set aside. Sauté the veggies in the pan using the fat from the meat. Beat the eggs in a bowl, then add the meat, veggies, cottage cheese, herbs and spices. Spoon into the muffin cups and sprinkle with the grated cheese. Cook for 15–20 minutes. Best served warm.

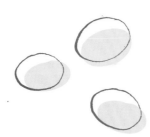

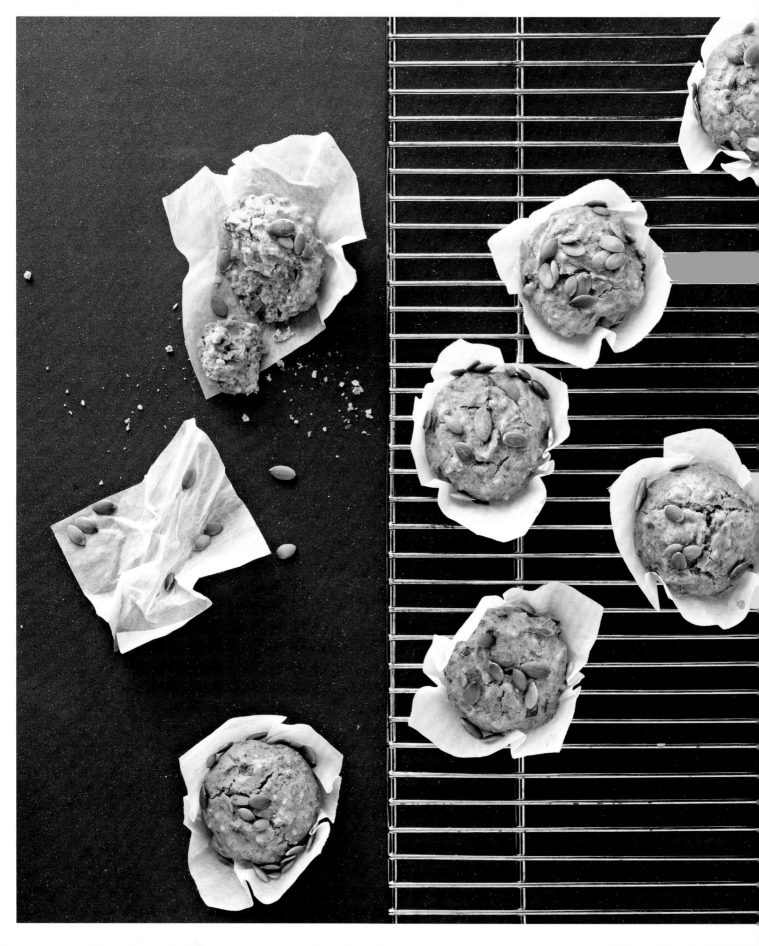

FLUFFY SQUASH AND CHIA MUFFINS

Trust me: these will work out. Don't worry about exact measurements, as long as the consistency is cakey. Bear in mind the chia seeds soak up stacks of liquid, so if you end up with a runny batter-like slop, add more chia seeds before spooning into the muffin pan. Get fancy and sprinkle the muffins with freshly torn basil and some flowers.

INGREDIENTS

½ cup butternut or kabocha squash

2 cups gluten-free flour (I use buckwheat and some chickpea flour)

1 cup almond meal

sprinkle of ground cinnamon

1 teaspoon baking powder

handful of basil leaves, chopped

fistful of chia seeds

2 eggs, separated

2–3 tablespoons granulated stevia

2 tablespoons olive oil

handful of pumpkin seeds

❄ **BATCH & FREEZE** ❘ **MAKES** 12–16

METHOD

Preheat the oven to 350°F and line each cup of a 12-cup muffin pan with a 4-inch square of baking paper (or use cupcake papers). Grate the squash using a food processor with a shredding disk—you need 1 cup grated squash. Combine the squash, flour, almond meal, cinnamon, baking powder, basil and chia seeds. In a separate bowl, beat the egg yolks, stevia and olive oil using an immersion blender, then add to the squash mixture. Stir in enough water to make a thick consistency (I use the immersion blender again for this). Whip the egg whites until soft peaks form and stir into the squash mixture. Spoon into the muffin cups and pop in the oven. After about 5 minutes, sprinkle the muffins with the pumpkin seeds. Bake for about 10 minutes. Serve warm or cold.

ZUCCHINI "CHEESECAKE"

This dish can also be jazzed up into a slightly special brunch meal.

INGREDIENTS

coconut oil or butter for greasing

2–3 large zucchini

1 teaspoon salt

15 ounces ricotta

¾ cup grated Parmesan

2 scallions, green parts only, chopped

2 cloves garlic, chopped

¼ cup chopped dill

zest of 1 lemon

2 large eggs, well beaten

⅓ cup crumbled feta

SERVES 8

METHOD

Preheat the oven to 325°F and grease a 9-in. cake pan or medium-sized baking dish. Grate the zucchini using a food processor with a shredding disk—you need 2 cups grated zucchini. Combine the zucchini and salt in a colander or sturdy sieve and let sit for 15 minutes, then use your fingers or a spoon to press out as much moisture as you can. Combine the ricotta, Parmesan, scallions, garlic, dill and lemon zest, then stir in the eggs and zucchini. Pour into the pan and bake for 1 hour. Sprinkle with the feta and return to the oven for 25 minutes or until the cheese has melted. The cake is best when left to cool completely so that it sets properly. Serve at room temperature.

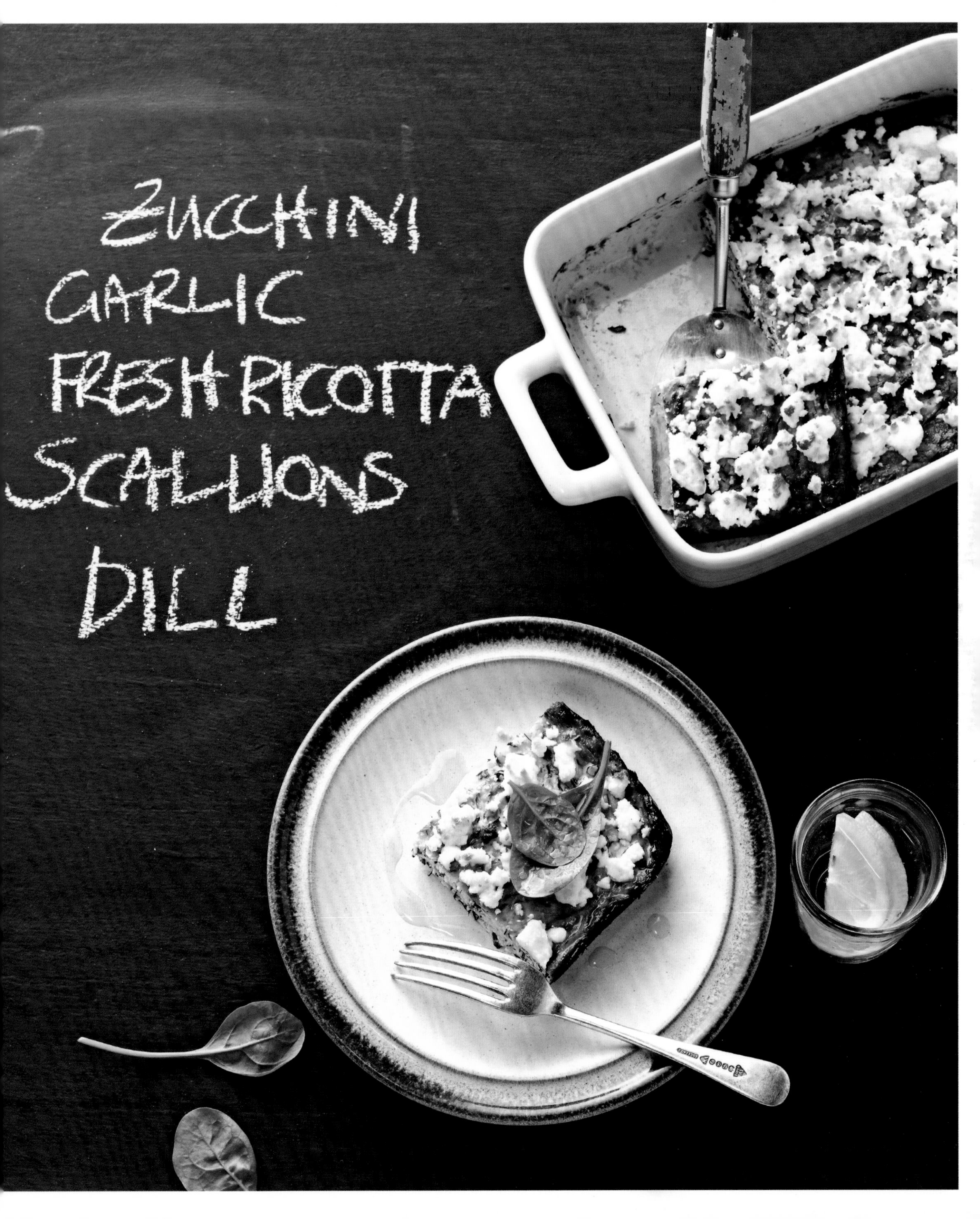

ZUCCHINI
GARLIC
FRESH RICOTTA
SCALLIONS
DILL

⇨ YES! SUGAR-FREE PANCAKES. HERE ARE THREE TYPES AND FIVE TOPPINGS THAT COVER ALL NEEDS AND TASTES. ⇦

The first is a great "Paleo" version and the third can be prepared as gluten free, too.

FIRST CHOOSE YOUR PANCAKE

COCONUT FLUFFS

INGREDIENTS

2 eggs, whisked

1¾ cups can coconut milk

2 tablespoons coconut oil or butter, melted, plus extra for frying

¼ cup coconut flour

¾ cup buckwheat flour

3 teaspoons baking powder

½ teaspoon salt

½ cup unsweetened shredded coconut

MAKES 4–6

METHOD

Combine the eggs, coconut milk and 2 tablespoons coconut oil. Stir in the remaining ingredients. Melt a generous dollop of butter or oil in a frying pan over medium–low heat. Pour in some batter. The mixture will make 4–6 large pancakes or 8–12 smaller ones. When the surface starts to bubble, flip and cook the other side. Repeat until all the batter is used.

⇨ turn over to page 100 for great mix-'n'-match toppings

SIMPLE APPLE PANCAKES

INGREDIENTS

1 cup self-rising flour
1 egg
1 cup milk
⅓ cup powdered stevia
1 apple, peeled and grated
butter for frying

MAKES 12

METHOD

Combine the flour, egg, milk and stevia, then add the apple and stir gently. Melt some butter in a frying pan over medium–low heat. Spoon in ⅓ cup batter. When the surface starts to bubble, flip and cook on the other side. Repeat until all the batter is used.

BUCKWHEAT GALETTES

INGREDIENTS

½ cup buckwheat flour
½ cup all-purpose flour
¼ teaspoon sea salt
1 egg
1 cup milk
2 tablespoons salted butter, melted, for greasing

MAKES 4–6

METHOD

Sift the flours and salt. Make a small well in the center. Whisk the egg and milk together in a small bowl, then pour into the well. Beat into a smooth batter the consistency of thick cream. Cover with plastic wrap and refrigerate for at least 2 hours or overnight. Remove the batter from the fridge and set aside for 20 minutes. Stir, adding 1–2 tablespoons of water if necessary. Heat a large non-stick frying pan over medium heat. Lightly grease the entire base of the pan with melted butter.

Add a small ladleful of batter and quickly swirl it around so you have a very thin layer covering the whole of the pan. Use a palette knife or spatula to spread out the mixture. Cook for 1 minute or until the galette comes away easily from the pan when you shake it. Flip the galette over and cook for 1–2 minutes. Repeat with the remaining batter.

NOTE

THE INCLUSION OF ALL-PURPOSE FLOUR IMPROVES THE TEXTURE OF THESE GALETTES. IF YOU WANT TO MAKE GLUTEN-FREE GALETTES, USE 1 CUP BUCKWHEAT FLOUR INSTEAD OF THE TWO FLOURS.

1

COCONUT BUTTER BOMB

Serve a pancake with a cube or two of Coconut Butter (see page 182), melted.

2

THE WALDORF

1 green apple, grated
lemon juice
1 cup homemade Cream Cheese (see page 64)
walnuts, preferably sprouted (see page 59)
½ cup brown rice syrup, heated
rock salt, to taste

Mix the apple with a little lemon juice to prevent it from browning. Place the cream cheese, apple and walnuts in separate bowls on the table and invite everyone to top their pancakes, starting with the cheese and then the walnuts, drizzling with a little syrup and sprinkling with rock salt.

3

SPICED BERRY SWIRL

Add a drizzle of Berry Grown-Up Sauce (see page 68) and a dollop of full-fat yogurt to your pancake and swirl a little.

4

SPICED PUMPKIN BUTTER AND PECANS

1 cup canned unsweetened pumpkin purée or Squash Purée (see page 58)
1 teaspoon ground cinnamon
½ teaspoon ground ginger
pinch of ground cloves (optional)
pinch of ground nutmeg (optional)
1 tablespoon brown rice syrup
1 tablespoon apple cider vinegar or lemon juice
knob of butter
½ cup pecans, preferably sprouted (see page 59) or Candied Pecans (see page 174)

Combine the squash purée, spices, syrup and ⅓ cup of water in a saucepan and bring to a boil. Reduce the heat and simmer for 30 minutes, stirring frequently. Stir in the vinegar and butter. Pour over the pancakes and sprinkle the pecans on top. The squash butter mixture will keep for 2 weeks, so feel free to make extra!

5
SO-FRENCHIE-SO-CHIC HAM AND CHEESE

6 slices ham
2 cups grated Gruyère or other cheese

This one only works with the Buckwheat Galettes (see page 99). Place a slice of ham and a large sprinkle of cheese in the center of each cooked galette and fold. I fold the galette in half, but you can do it as a "pouch" or in quarters. Heat in a frying pan until the cheese melts.

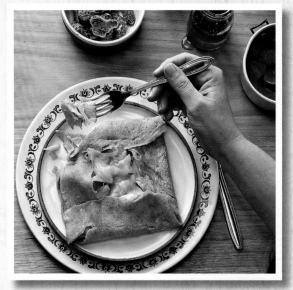

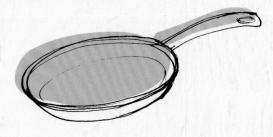

Coconut butter—melt a few down for an instant coconut butter bomb.

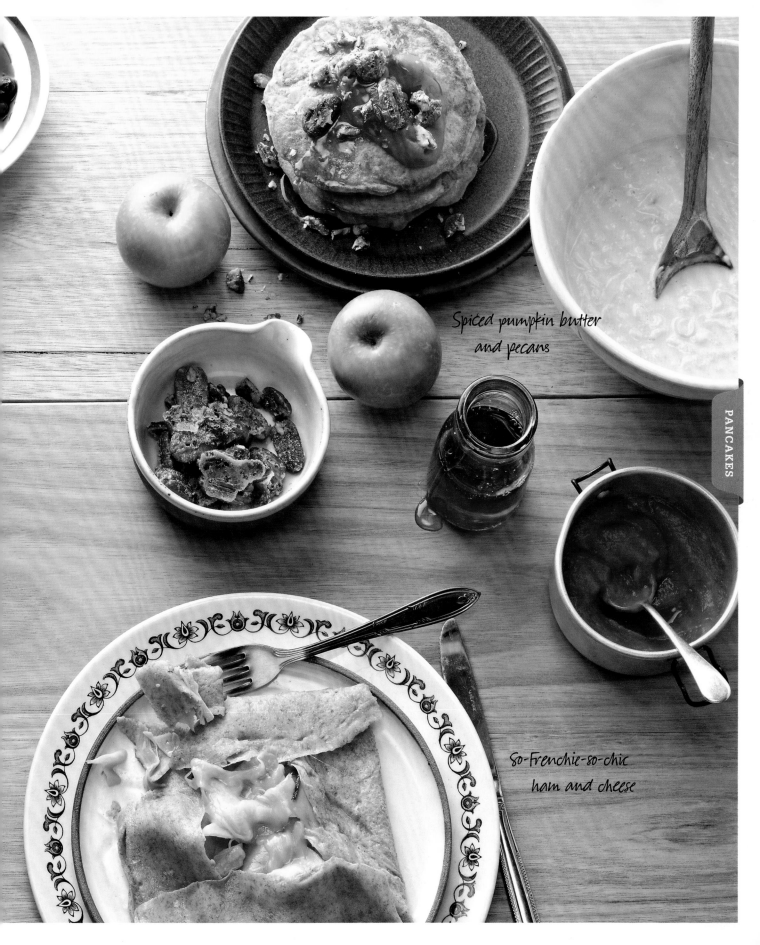

Spiced pumpkin butter and pecans

So-Frenchie-so-chic ham and cheese

BREAKFAST CASSEROLE

I love the idea of a breakfast casserole—it breaks so many rules (turnips
for breakfast?!). I like to keep it simple and use one vegetable at a time.
Turnips, rutabagas or sweet potato work best for this recipe, in my opinion. This
is also a good way to use up random sausages left in the fridge after a barbeque.
You can double the recipe and place half the mixture in another baking dish,
cover and freeze to cook the following week.

INGREDIENTS

coconut oil or butter for greasing
3 turnips, peeled (or 2 rutabagas or 1 large
sweet potato)
2 sausages or a large handful of ground pork or beef
3 scallions, green parts only, chopped
4 eggs, beaten

❄ **BATCH & FREEZE** | **SERVES** 4

METHOD

Preheat the oven to 375°F and grease a small
glass or ceramic baking dish. Grate the turnips,
using a food processor if you have one. If using
sausages, remove the meat and discard the
casings. Brown the meat with a little oil in a large
hot frying pan until not quite cooked through,
breaking it up into small pieces with a spoon
or spatula. Toss in the rest of the ingredients and
stir, then spoon into the baking dish. Bake for
45 minutes. Let it stand for a few minutes so the
casserole sets before you cut into it. Serve warm.

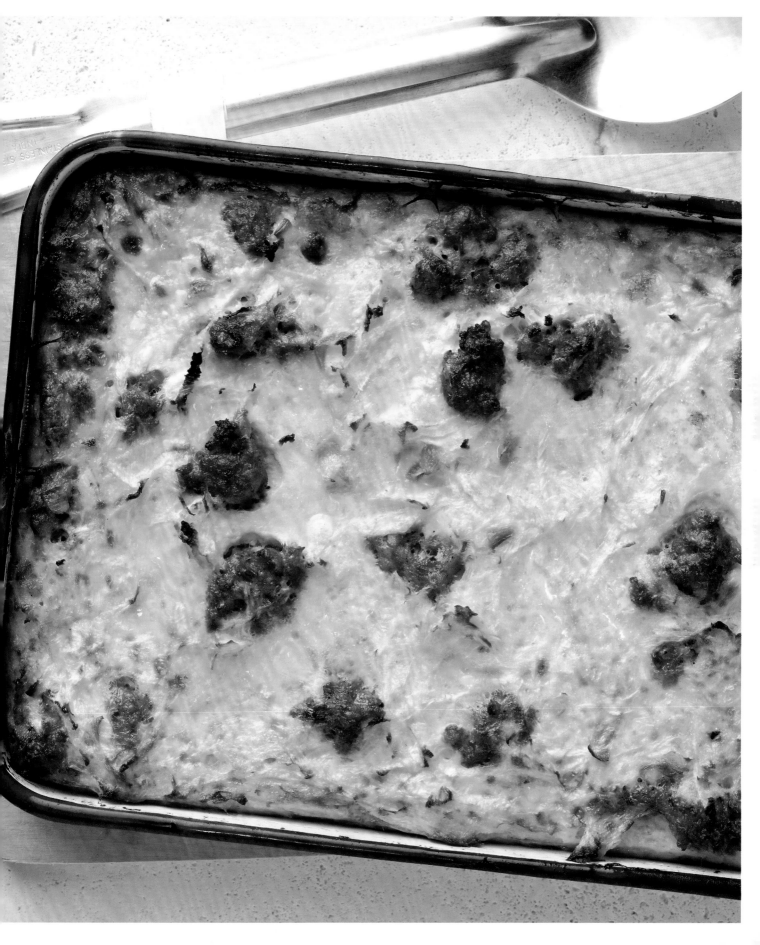

POLENTA PATTIES WITH SAUTÉED GREENS, POACHED EGGS AND ROMA TOMATO BASIL SALSA

Dr. Rob Lustig is the medical High Priest of the sugar-free movement having committed much of his career to studying the real causes of obesity (and—oh, hello— finding sugar is the culprit). His fervor has often given me courage in my own journey and we've recently become e-mates, sharing ideas and links to new research. I'm super grateful for his insights! Ergo, I'm super thrilled he and his recipe developer Cindy Gershen have kindly shared this lovely brunch dish with me from his new *The Fat Chance Cookbook*.

INGREDIENTS

4 cups water

salt to taste

1 cup corn grits or cornmeal

2 tablespoons olive oil, plus more for pan

6 cups greens: spinach, chard, or kale, rinsed

6 eggs

½ cup Roma Tomato Basil Salsa

ROMA TOMATO BASIL SALSA

1 pound Roma tomatoes, diced into ¼-inch pieces

1 tablespoon minced garlic

½ cup chopped fresh basil

½ cup extra-virgin olive oil

¼ cup apple cider vinegar

1 tablespoon cracked black pepper

1 teaspoon salt

SERVES 6

METHOD

To make the polenta, bring the water and salt to a boil in a large pot over high heat. Slowly add the grits, whisking constantly to keep lumps from forming. When the mixture is smooth, reduce the heat to low and simmer gently for 30 minutes, until very thick. Stir occasionally to keep the polenta from sticking. The polenta should have the consistency of mashed potatoes. Oil an 8-by-8-in. pan and pour the polenta into the pan to cool until firm.

Remove the polenta from the loaf pan and cut 6 slices, each ¼ inch thick.

Heat 1 tablespoon of the olive oil in a large pan over medium-high heat. Add the polenta slices and fry until golden brown on both sides, about 3 minutes per side.

Add the remaining 1 tablespoon of oil to the pan, and sauté the greens until wilted and tender.

Place a polenta patty on each of 6 plates. Top each patty with greens. Place the eggs on top.

Poach the eggs (see page 84).

Mix the salsa ingredients together in a bowl. This will make 2 cups. Pour a few tablespoons of salsa over each egg. Reserve the remaining salsa for other uses.

COCONUT CURRY MEATBALLS

I love most of the recipes by Mark at his Mark's Daily Apple website, but this one he's shared with me is a standout! Mark says: "You can buy pre-ground chicken if you like, but it takes hardly any time to grind it yourself in a food processor. A combination of thigh and breast meat yields a moist meatball that will hold together well."

INGREDIENTS

1½ lbs. skinless chicken fillets

1 carrot, grated

2 cloves garlic

½ cup unsweetened shredded coconut

1 egg

2 teaspoons curry powder

½ teaspoon salt

handful of cilantro or flat-leaf parsley leaves, to taste

coconut or olive oil

MAKES 24

METHOD

Put everything except the oil in the food processor and blend until smooth. Using your hands, form 24 small balls (smaller balls cook quicker). Heat several tablespoons of oil in a large frying pan over medium–high heat. When it is hot enough that a meatball sizzles as soon as it hits the pan, put the meatballs in. You might have to cook these in batches. Cook for 2 minutes, then roll the meatballs over and cook for 5 minutes more. Put a lid on the pan and cook for another 6–8 minutes. Serve immediately.

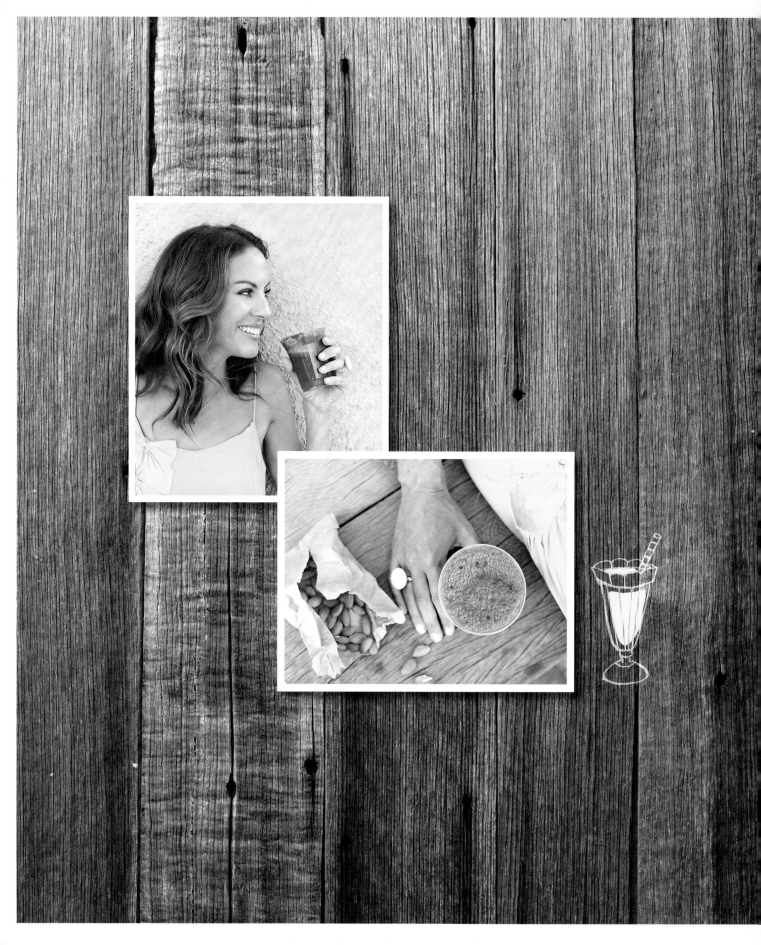

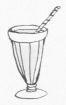

SMOOTHIES & DRINKS

The smoothies I share here with you cut to the chase—they are full of nutrition, quick to make and a convenient way of using supplements to repair the balance in your stomach and your digestive system lining: antioxidant powders, green powders, slippery elm powder, chia seeds and so on. The hot drinks are designed for sugar-free comfort and joy.

TIPS FOR: SMOOTH SMOOTHIES

- If a recipe contains coconut oil, always add it just before you blend so it doesn't turn solid in the cold liquid. During the winter months you may have to melt the coconut oil on a gentle heat before you put it in.
- Put all the ingredients in a wide drinking glass and mix using an immersion blender. This is a great way to save on equipment.
- Remember to always use full-fat dairy in your smoothies. (See page 28 to remind yourself of why.)
- If you have to eat on the run, add extra chia seeds and ice and place the smoothie in the freezer for a few minutes to set (so it doesn't spill).

SWEET GREEN MEAL-IN-A-TUMBLER

This recipe evolved out of necessity. I wanted a green drink for those days when I knew I wouldn't be eating as well as I'd like, and that could travel (i.e., wouldn't spill). The grapefruit and chia make this really thick, while the green powder adds a nutritional kick and "sweetness."

INGREDIENTS

½ grapefruit
½ lemon
½ green apple
1 cucumber
handful of lettuce, arugula or watercress
handful of mint or cilantro leaves
1 teaspoon chia seeds
2 teaspoons green powder
½ to 1 cup coconut water
handful of ice

SERVES 1–3

METHOD

If you're using a high-powered blender, toss all the ingredients in together—seeds and all—and blend for a minute or so. This will make 2–3 servings.

If you're using a juicer, juice the grapefruit, lemon, apple, cucumber, lettuce and herbs, then stir in the remaining ingredients. This will make 1–2 servings.

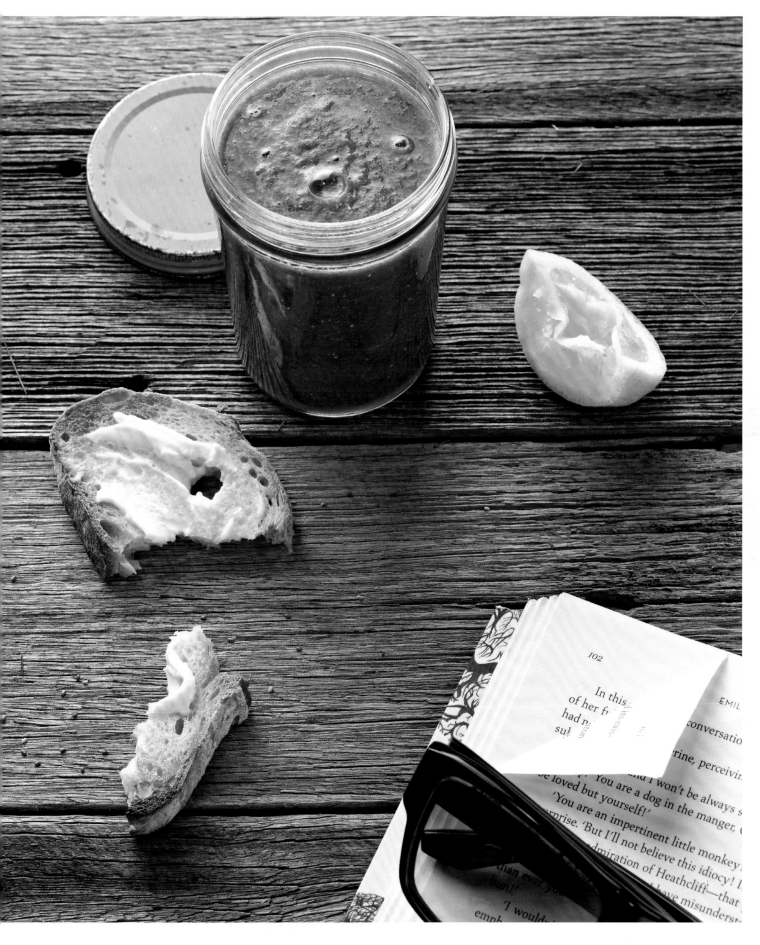

SPINACH AND FENNEL SMOOTHIE

My friend Joe Cross (who made the eye-opening documentary *Fat, Sick and Nearly Dead*) shares this fruit-free digestive number.

INGREDIENTS

1 bulb fennel
1 cucumber
3 stalks celery
3 cups baby spinach leaves
handful of ice (optional)
splash coconut water (optional)

SERVES 2 OR 3

METHOD

Throw all the ingredients into a high-powered blender and blend until smooth.

MAKE-ME-OVER MOJITO SMOOTHIE

INGREDIENTS

1 cup coconut water
juice of 2 limes
1 small ripe avocado
handful of mint leaves
small handful of baby spinach leaves (optional)
pinch of vanilla powder
pinch of powdered stevia
1–2 teaspoons spirulina powder or 2 tablespoons green powder
small handful of ice cubes

SERVES 2

METHOD

Throw all the ingredients into a blender and blend until smooth.

BERRY YOGURT SMOOTHIE

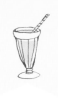

INGREDIENTS

1 cup full-fat organic plain yogurt

1 egg

small handful of frozen mixed berries

½ teaspoon ground cinnamon

small pinch of granulated stevia

1 teaspoon chia seeds

1 tablespoon coconut oil

SERVES 2 OR 3

METHOD

Throw all the ingredients into a blender (add the coconut oil last so it doesn't turn solid in the cold yogurt) and blend until smooth.

ICED LEMONGRASS AND GINGER ZING

One of the best sugar-craving fixes is making a cup of tea. It can distract you for 5 minutes—enough time for the yen to pass—and can calm you and restore some gentle steadiness. Muriel Barbery writes in her philosophically delicate novel *The Elegance of the Hedgehog*: "Yes, the world may aspire to vacuousness, insignificance surrounds us. Then let us drink a cup of tea. Silence descends."

INGREDIENTS

1 tablespoon ground lemongrass

1 tablespoon ground ginger

MAKES 1 POT

METHOD

Make up a pot of tea using the lemongrass and ginger. Let cool, then place in the fridge. It will brew further in the fridge. Strain to serve.

CHOCOLATE CHIP AND MINT WHIP

INGREDIENTS

1⅔ cups homemade Almond Milk (see page 65)

1 small ripe avocado

large handful of mint leaves

3 tablespoons organic whey-based
protein powder (optional)

2 tablespoons green powder (optional)

1–2 generous pinches powdered stevia, to taste

small handful of ice cubes

2 tablespoons cacao nibs

MAKES 2

METHOD

Throw all the ingredients, except the cacao nibs, into a blender and blend until smooth. Toss in the nibs and blend for an extra few pulses.

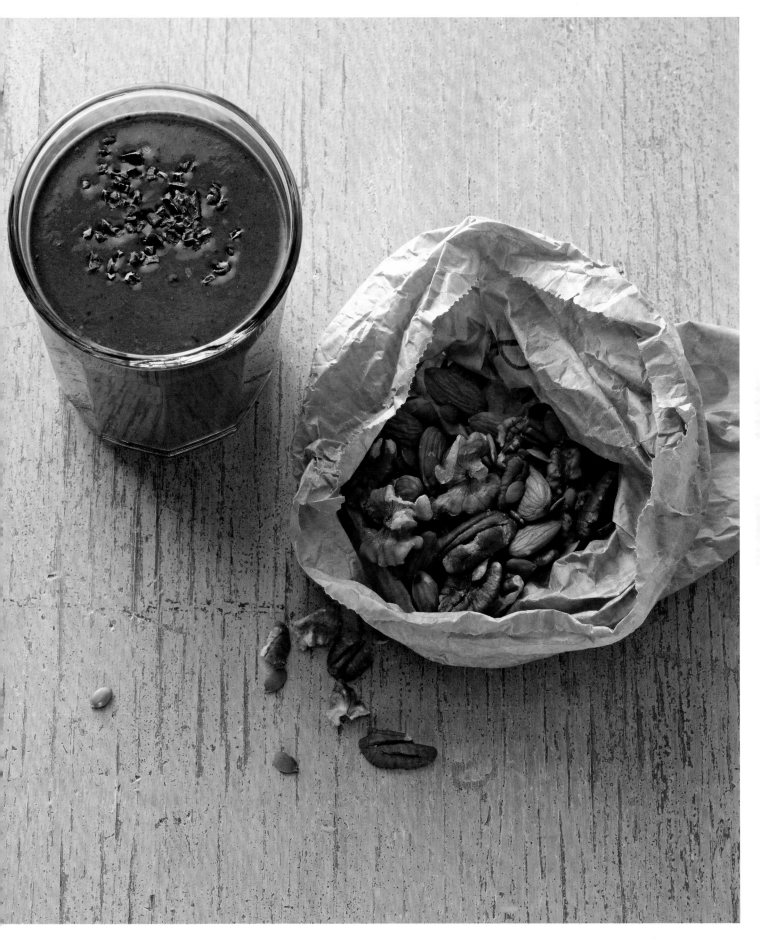

We shot this iced chai with the raw beans because, well, I'm known to eat raw vegetables at odd times!

ROOIBOS CHAI

This is a wonderfully nourishing version of the standard black tea chai. Rooibos is easy to find at most health-food shops and even at supermarkets. The spices used in this blend are perfect for curbing an afternoon sweet craving—the licorice provides a sweet kick while killing the blood-sugar craziness. You can also make this with regular black tea or dandelion root, if you prefer.

INGREDIENTS

3 cardamom pods

3 cloves

3 peppercorns

3 star anise or 1 teaspoon fennel seeds

1-in. piece fresh ginger, finely chopped (I leave the skin on), or 1 tablespoon ground ginger

1 teaspoon ground licorice root (optional; see Resources, page 205)

1 cup milk or homemade Almond Milk (see page 65)

¼ cup loose organic rooibos tea

SERVES 4

METHOD

Using a mortar and pestle, lightly crush the cardamom, cloves, peppercorns and star anise (alternatively, leave them whole). Transfer the crushed spices to a saucepan and add the ginger, licorice root (if using) and 3 cups water. Bring to a boil, then reduce the heat and simmer for 4 minutes. Take the saucepan off the heat and let steep for 4–5 minutes. Add the milk and rooibos tea and bring back to a boil. Remove from the heat, cover and steep for another 5 minutes. Strain and serve.

TRY THESE DELICIOUS VARIATIONS:

- To make an iced version, omit the milk and place the chai in the fridge overnight to steep further. Strain the concentrate, then serve over ice with cold milk.

- To make a mocha chai version, stir in 2 tablespoons raw cacao powder at the end.

- For a super-fun treat, blend the strained hot milky chai with 4 tablespoons almond butter.

CHOCOLATE PEANUT BUTTER HOT COCOA

Angela at Oh She Glows vegan blog chose this hot beverage for us. It's wintry indulgent goodness in a cup!

INGREDIENTS

1¾ cups can coconut milk
½ cup homemade Almond Milk (see page 65)
⅔ cup brown rice syrup, or to taste
2 tablespoons natural peanut butter
½ cup raw cacao powder, sifted well
pinch of salt, or to taste
cacao nibs to garnish (optional)

SERVES 2 OR 3

METHOD

Throw all the ingredients except the cacao nibs into a saucepan and whisk like crazy. Bring to a low boil, then simmer for several minutes while whisking to remove any remaining clumps. Pour into mugs and top with cacao nibs to serve, if you like.

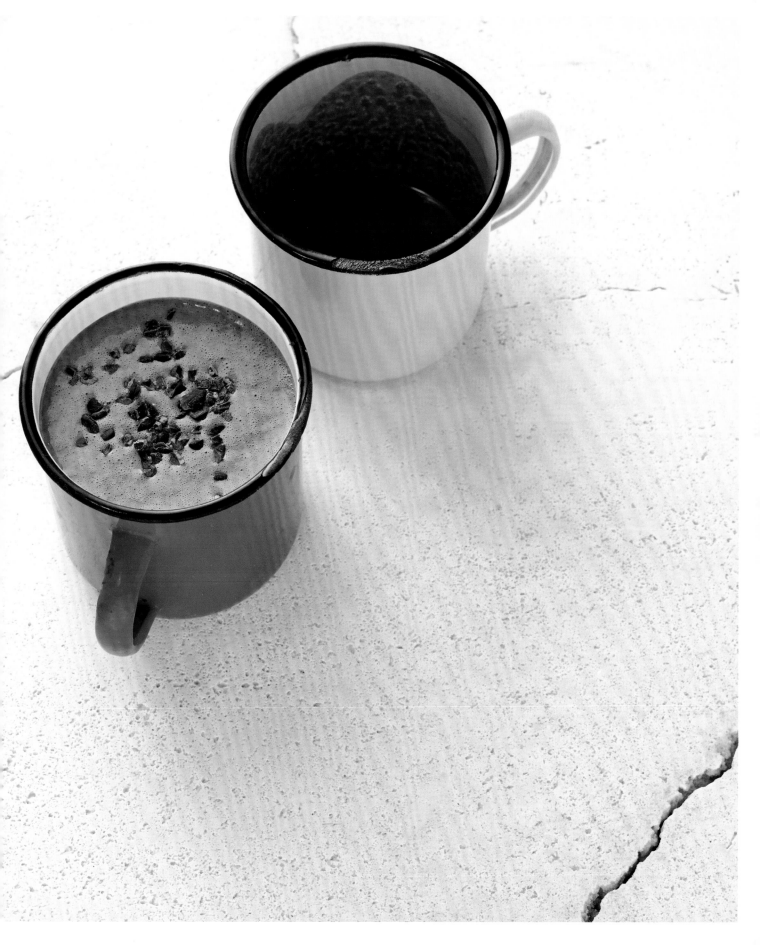

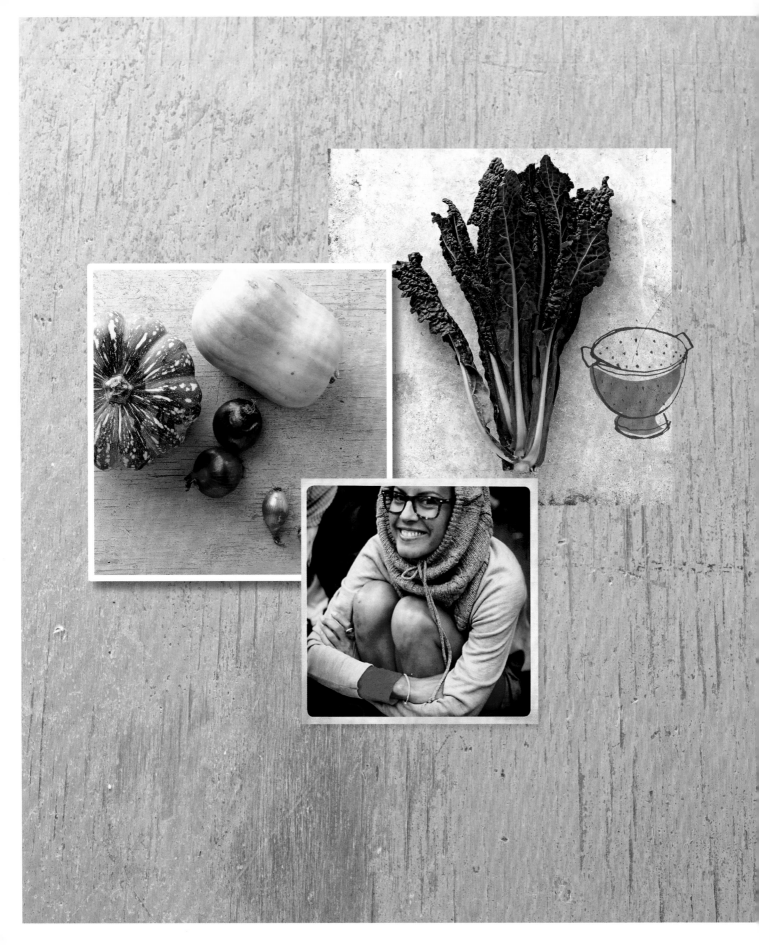

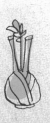

HEALTHY DETOX MEALS

⇨ FOR THE SUGAR DETOX PERIOD AND BEYOND ⇦

As you know, one of my main good-eating tricks is to "crowd out"—that is, eat as much nutritious, good stuff as you can and then see if you still want something sweet.

This approach ensures I'm primed with nutrition when I make the conscious choice to indulge or not.

It also means I'm giving my body the best chance of being able to recalibrate and balance itself, which really is key when you go through the initial sugar detox period. The meals in this section all incorporate ingredients that are alkalizing, cooling and detoxing. Dose up on one or three of these a day and you'll feel energized and balanced—no sugar required.

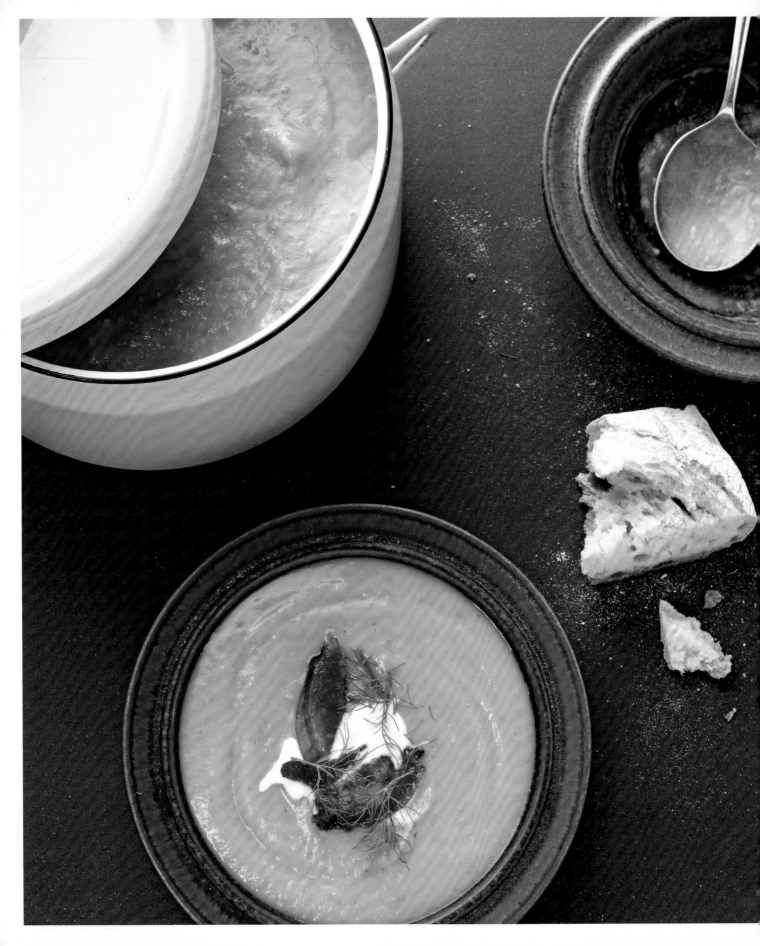

FOOLPROOF FENNEL SOUP

This soup is both green and sweet. It reminds me of my mum. She's not green, but she's definitely sweet and she used to cook with fennel and red potatoes a lot when I was younger. She's also a big soup fan. It's where I got it from.

INGREDIENTS

5 tablespoons butter

2 large fennel bulbs, sliced (reserve the leaves for garnish)

2 leeks, sliced

2 teaspoons fennel seeds (or a mixture of fennel and anise seeds and ground licorice root)

splash of apple cider vinegar or white wine

6 cups Basic Chicken Stock (see page 60)

2 garlic cloves, chopped

2 red potatoes, chopped (or 1 cup leftover cooked rice)

yogurt or sour cream or shaved Parmesan, to serve

4 slices pancetta, fried until crisp, cooled and crumbled

pinch of salt

❄ **BATCH & FREEZE** ❘ **SERVES** 4

METHOD

Melt the butter in a large saucepan. Sauté the fennel and leeks until soft, then add the fennel seeds. Add the vinegar, stir a little, and pour in the stock. Bring to the boil. Add the garlic and potatoes, then cover and simmer for 30 minutes. Remove from the heat and blend using an immersion blender. Serve the soup with a dollop of yogurt or sour cream or some shaved Parmesan, sprinkled with the crumbled pancetta, snipped fennel leaves and a pinch of salt.

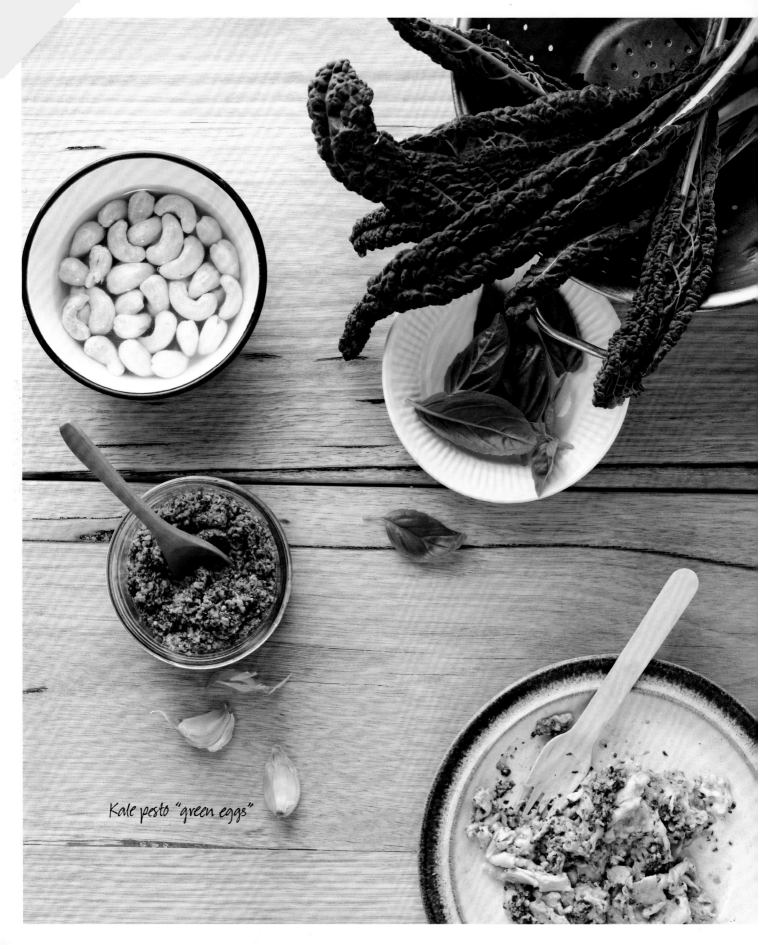

Kale pesto "green eggs"

FOUR TASTY PESTOS

➡ PESTO IS A WONDERFUL WAY TO GET GREENS INTO YOUR DIET. IT'S ALSO EASY TO MAKE AND CAN BE PREPARED IN BULK SO IT'S READY TO ADD TO YOUR MEAL. HERE, I'VE CREATED FOUR LUSH FLAVOR BOMBS, PLUS SOME FRESH WAYS TO EAT THEM! ⬅

Many pesto recipes call for pine nuts, but I tend to use cashews because pine nuts are quite fragile and can go rancid quickly. In all these recipes you can choose to use Parmesan, nuts or a combination of both, but if you omit the Parmesan, add a little extra salt. If you have some spinach or arugula leaves, feel free to add them to any of the recipes to add extra green love. Each recipe makes 1½ cups.

CILANTRO PESTO

Fresh cilantro is an herb that is a great natural detoxifier and is anti-inflammatory. Ditto the cayenne pepper.

2 cups cilantro leaves
2 medium scallions, green parts only
2 cloves garlic
3 tablespoons olive oil
juice of 1 lime
¼ cup grated Parmesan or ½ cup cashews, soaked in water for 1–4 hours and drained
¼ teaspoon cayenne pepper
salt and freshly ground black pepper, to taste

Place all the ingredients in a food processor or blender and process until creamy and smooth. Store in a sealed container in the fridge for up to 1 week, or cover with a layer of oil and freeze.

BROCCOLI PESTO

2 cups broccoli florets
2 medium scallions, green parts only
2 cloves garlic
3 tablespoons olive oil
juice of 1 lemon
¼ cup grated Parmesan or ½ cup cashews, soaked in water for 1–4 hours and drained
salt and freshly ground black pepper, to taste

Steam the broccoli florets. Place all the ingredients in a food processor or blender and process until creamy and smooth. Store in a sealed container in the fridge for up to 1 week, or cover with a layer of oil and freeze.

PESTO

KALE PESTO

Note: I prefer this one with Parmesan instead of nuts.

1 medium bunch kale, stems removed
2 medium scallions, green parts only
2 cloves garlic
3 tablespoons olive oil
juice of 1 lemon
¼ cup grated Parmesan
salt and freshly ground black pepper, to taste

Steam the kale leaves for 2–3 minutes. Place all the ingredients in a food processor or blender and process until creamy and smooth. Store in a sealed container in the fridge for up to 1 week, or cover with a layer of oil and freeze.

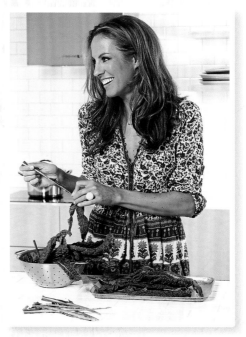

BASIL PESTO

I prefer cashews in my basil pesto as they temper the flavor best. I use ½ cup cashews in this recipe, but you can make a less creamy version by reducing the quantity of cashews.

½ cup cashews, soaked in water for 1–4 hours
    and drained
2 medium scallions, green parts only
2 garlic cloves
2 cups basil leaves
3 tablespoons olive oil
juice of 1 lemon
salt and freshly ground black pepper, to taste

Blend all the ingredients in a food processor or blender until smooth. Store in a sealed container in the fridge for up to 1 week, or cover with a layer of oil and freeze.

TIP

Want to know how to remove kale stalks? Grab the stalk end and then run your fingers down it in one fluid motion to shear off the leaf. Keep the stalks in the freezer to use in stocks (see page 60).

1

BROCCOLI PESTO QUINOA

½ cup broccoli florets
dash of heavy cream or ½ ripe avocado
⅓ cup broccoli pesto (see page 125)
½ cup cooked quinoa (see page 61) or pasta
olive oil, lemon juice and crumbled feta, to serve

Steam the broccoli florets. Add the cream to the broccoli pesto and blend briefly until creamy and smooth. Toss the quinoa and broccoli florets with most of the broccoli pesto. To serve, pour some oil over the top, add extra broccoli pesto and a squeeze of lemon juice, and sprinkle with feta.

2

PESTO AND GOAT'S CHEESE DIP

Mix pesto with goat's cheese or homemade Cream Cheese (see page 64) to make a dip.

3

PESTO FISH

Dollop a spoonful of pesto on grilled white fish.

4

FANCY VEGGIES

Sauté pesto with vegetables such as Brussels sprouts or asparagus.

5

PESTO SANDWICHES

Spread pesto on rice cakes or toast with a slice of tomato, ham, cheese and zucchini.

6

GREEN EGGS

Add pesto to scrambled eggs (see page 87).

PESTO

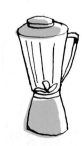

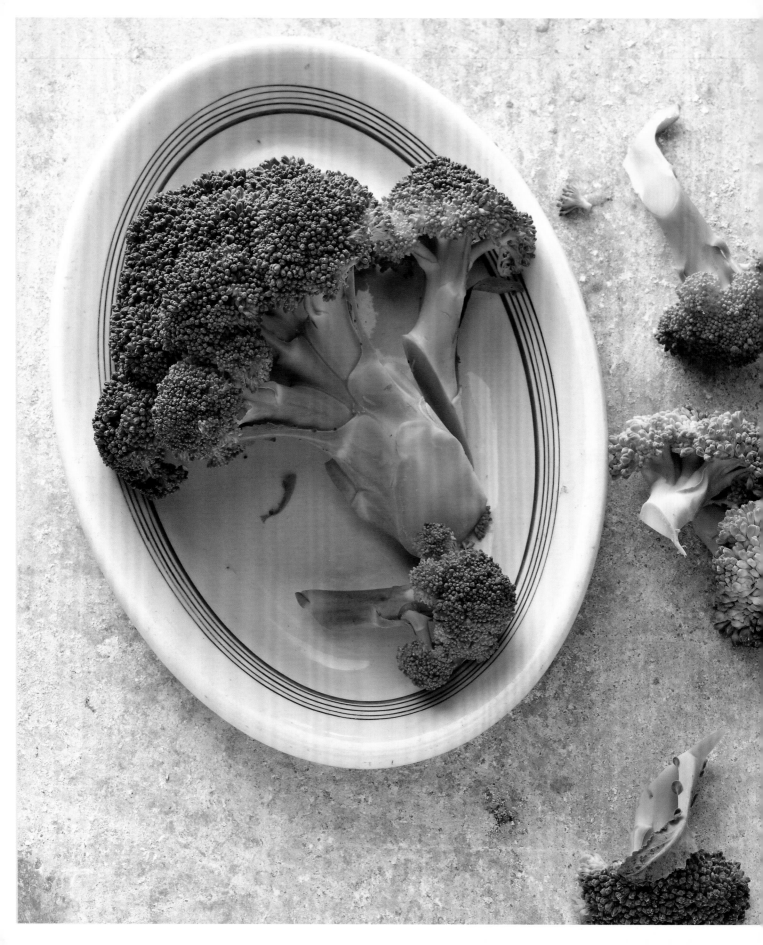

CHEESY GREEN MISH-MASH SOUP

The best thing about this soup is you don't have to try at all. It's great for using up vegetables that are lying around. Oh, and kids love it. Don't bother cutting the vegetables too precisely and don't worry if you only have, say, broccoli in the fridge— it's all good. Just get the green goodness in and life flows from there. Having said that, a combination of zucchini and broccoli works best. Throw in some celery, too, if you have it, including the leaves.

INGREDIENTS

3 tablespoons coconut oil or butter

1 onion, roughly chopped

2 cloves garlic, chopped

6 cups roughly chopped green vegetables (zucchini, broccoli, celery—whatever you have)

4 cups vegetable stock or Basic Chicken Stock (see page 60)

1 cup arugula or watercress (optional)

1 cup roughly chopped cilantro, basil or flat-leaf parsley leaves

pinch of salt

juice of 1 lemon

½ cup crumbled sharp Cheddar

❄ **BATCH & FREEZE** | **SERVES** 6

METHOD

In a large saucepan, over medium-low heat, melt the coconut oil and sauté the onion and garlic. Add the green vegetables and stir for a minute, then pour in the stock and bring to a boil. Reduce the heat and simmer for 10–15 minutes. Stir in the arugula, herbs and salt. Turn off the heat and purée until smooth using an immersion blender, or transfer to a blender and pulse. Whisk in the lemon juice and stir in the cheese. Serve hot.

VARIATIONS

Instead of the cheese, serve the soup with a dollop of yogurt or sour cream and a drizzle of olive oil.

➥ I LOVE MAKING A HASH OF MY LUNCH. WHAT'S A HASH MEAL? IT'S A WAY OF COOKING AND EATING THAT I VERY MUCH SUBSCRIBE TO. HASHES ARE ABOUT WORKING WITH THE DENSELY NUTRITIOUS INGREDIENTS YOU HAVE IN THE FRIDGE (OR FREEZER) AND TOSSING THEM TOGETHER IN TASTY WAYS. HASHES ARE ALL ABOUT EFFICIENCY, SUSTAINABILITY AND HEIGHTENED FLAVOR. ➥

For me hash meals entail mixing up leftovers—meat, beans, vegetables—from the night before, frying them with some cheese and/or an egg, and tossing through fresh herbs for zing. I also like to squeeze a lemon over, to cut through any saturated flavors.

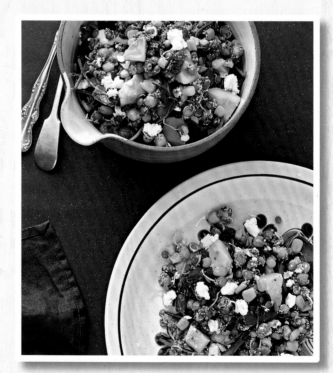

NOTE

You'll notice that I don't provide precise quantities for these recipes. I use a handful of this or that, or whatever I've got. I suggest you do the same! It's a great opportunity to play and get a little bit loose. You have permission!

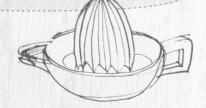

One of my favorite vitamin bombs: warm sprouted pea hash

SQUASH AND PUMPKIN SEED HASH

INGREDIENTS

butternut or kabocha squash, chopped into 1 in. chunks

salt

coconut oil

frozen peas

parcooked-and-frozen broccoli (see page 59)

ground cinnamon

pumpkin seeds

unsweetened coconut flakes or unsweetened shredded coconut

yogurt

METHOD

Sauté the squash and salt in coconut oil in a pan. Add the peas and broccoli, cooking for a few minutes until they have thawed and heated through, then add cinnamon. Transfer to a serving bowl. Toss the pumpkin seeds in the same pan and add the coconut right at the end (it toasts super-fast) and cook until golden. Blob some yogurt onto the vegetable mixture and scatter the coconut and pumpkin seeds on top.

WARM SPROUTED PEA HASH

INGREDIENTS

sprouted legumes (see page 65)

dash of Basic Chicken Stock (see page 60)

or liquid aminos (see Resources, page 205)

chopped anchovies

crumbled feta

baby spinach leaves

avocado chunks

chia seeds (optional)

frozen corn kernels (optional)

METHOD

Sauté the sprouted legumes in a little chicken stock (use a block or three from the ice-cube tray, if you have some) and a dash of water. Add the anchovies, then the feta and spinach. Toss quickly to wilt the spinach a little. Add the remaining ingredients, remove from the heat and serve.

TIP

I toss chia seeds through many of these kinds of meals. They soak up any excess liquid and make the meal seem weightier. They also add instant protein and fiber.

MUSHROOM HASH

INGREDIENTS
sliced mushrooms
shaved ham, torn up
eggs, lightly beaten (1–2 per person)
milk
chia seeds

METHOD
Sauté the mushrooms and ham in a frying pan until both turn golden, then swirl through some beaten egg, a splash of milk and the chia seeds. Gently stir until the mixture forms a bit of a scramble, then serve.

TURMERIC, BROCCOLI ANTI-INFLAMMATORY HASH

Feeling a bit blah? Toxic? The greenery and turmeric in this meal will bring things back in balance.

INGREDIENTS
chopped red onion
parcooked-and-frozen broccoli (see page 59)
sprouted legumes (optional; see page 65)
1–2 cubes frozen Basic Chicken Stock (see page 60)
or 1–2 teaspoons oil
a little grated fresh turmeric or turmeric paste
(grated turmeric preserved in apple cider vinegar)
or ground turmeric
eggs (1–2 per person)
1 avocado

METHOD
Sauté the onion, broccoli and sprouted legumes in the chicken stock. Stir in the turmeric, then toss through an egg or two, stirring to break up the yolks and disperse it through the vegetables. Once the white starts to firm, stir through the avocado (to warm it). Serve.

SAUSAGE, WALNUT AND BEET HASH

INGREDIENTS

1 good-quality sausage (I like a pork sausage
with fennel seeds)

1 small parcooked-and-frozen beet (see page 59), cut
into ½-in. cubes, or wedges

red onion or a few green shallots

a few kale leaves, de-veined and finely chopped

splash of apple cider vinegar

handful walnuts, preferably sprouted (see page 59)

yogurt and olive oil, to serve

finely chopped preserved lemon (optional), to serve

METHOD

Cook the sausage in a frying pan until almost
done. Remove and chop into 1-in. chunks, then set
aside. Add the beet, onion and kale to the pan and
sauté. Add a little vinegar and stir, scraping any
cooked bits from the bottom of the pan. Cook for
3–5 minutes, until the kale is soft. Return the
sausage to the pan and add the walnuts. Serve with
yogurt and a little oil drizzled over, or combine
some preserved lemon, oil and yogurt and spoon
on top.

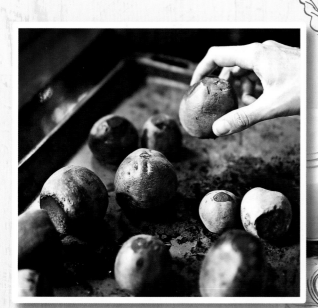

TIP
If you don't have kale, you can use
beet leaves instead.

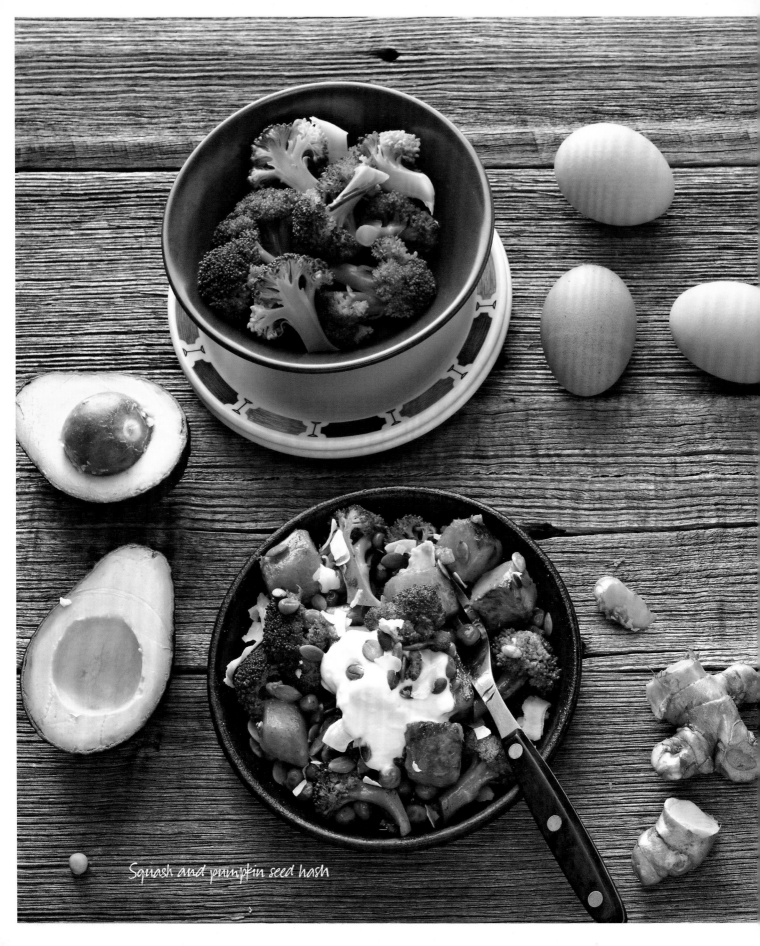

Squash and pumpkin seed hash

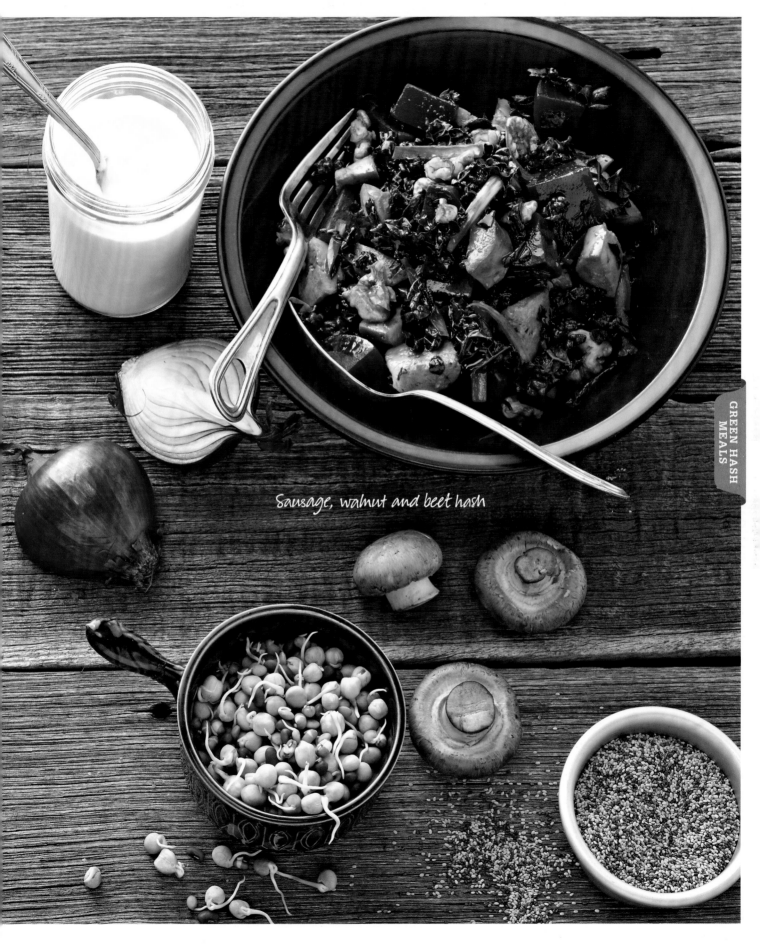

Sausage, walnut and beet hash

ROASTED CAULIFLOWER AND LEEK SOUP WITH DANDELION GREENS AND HAZELNUT PESTO

This very pretty soup and accompanying muffins (opposite) come as gifts from my beautiful "virtual" pal Aran Goyoaga. This nutrient-dense soup is her favorite and I adore these muffins, which we workshopped to become fructose-free. Go ahead and make a big batch and eat them as a meal unto themselves. P.S. Aran likes to use dandelion greens in her pesto as they're "among the most nutritious leafy greens you can find." But if you can't get a hold of some, use kale or arugula.

DANDELION AND GREEN HAZELNUT PESTO

¾ cup hazelnuts

1 clove garlic, minced

2 cups dandelion greens

2 tablespoons grated Parmesan cheese

½ teaspoon salt

¼ cup olive oil

ROASTED CAULIFLOWER AND LEEK SOUP

1 medium cauliflower (1 pound), cut into small florets

½ medium leek, cut into large rings

1 medium yellow onion, diced

2 garlic cloves, peeled

2 tablespoons olive oil

1½ teaspoons salt

¼ teaspoon freshly ground black pepper

1 medium russet potato, peeled and diced

2 cups Basic Chicken Stock (see page 60)

½ cup coconut milk

1 teaspoon fresh thyme leaves

SERVES 4 to 6

METHOD

To make the pesto, place the hazelnuts in a dry skillet and toast over medium-high heat for 5 minutes, until golden. Transfer to a dry kitchen towel and rub together to remove their skins. Combine the garlic and hazelnuts in a food processor and process to a fine powder. Add the dandelion greens, Parmesan and salt and continue processing. Add the olive oil in a single stream while the machine is running until the ingredients come together into a creamy paste. The pesto may be stored in the refrigerator for up to 3 days or frozen for up to 1 month.

To make the soup, preheat the oven to 375°F. Toss together the cauliflower, leek, onion, garlic, olive oil and ½ teaspoon of the salt. Transfer to a baking sheet and roast for 25 minutes, until golden. Then place the roasted vegetables in a large pot. Add the potato, chicken stock, coconut milk, thyme leaves, remaining 1 teaspoon salt and the pepper. Bring the liquid to a boil over medium-high heat. Reduce the heat to medium, cover and simmer for 10 minutes, until all the vegetables are tender. Purée the soup in a blender.

Serve with the pesto and the Squash, Apple and Blue Cheese Muffins (opposite).

SQUASH, APPLE AND
BLUE CHEESE MUFFINS

INGREDIENTS

1 cup superfine brown rice flour

½ cup millet flour

¼ cup potato starch

1 teaspoon baking powder

½ teaspoon baking soda

¼ teaspoon salt

1 tablespoon finely chopped fresh sage leaves

1 teaspoon fresh thyme leaves

1 cup canned, unsweetened pumpkin purée or Squash
Purée (page 58)

1 egg, lightly beaten

¼ cup brown rice syrup

¼ cup olive oil

2 ounces blue cheese, crumbled

1 medium Gala apple, peeled, cored and grated

MAKES 12 muffins

METHOD

Preheat the oven to 350°F. In a large bowl, whisk together the rice flour, millet flour, potato starch, baking powder, baking soda, salt, sage and thyme leaves. Add the pumpkin purée, egg, brown rice syrup and olive oil. Whisk until combined. Fold in the blue cheese and grated apple, juice and all. It will be a thick batter, similar to a soft scone dough. Scoop the batter into a muffin pan lined with baking papers. Bake for 18 to 20 minutes, until golden brown. Let the muffins cool in the pan for 5 minutes, and then transfer to a cooling rack.

They will keep for 3 days in an airtight container, or they can be frozen for up to 1 month.

COOLING AVOCADO SOUP

INGREDIENTS

1 large ripe avocado or 2 small ripe avocados, roughly chopped

2 small cucumbers, roughly chopped

1 scallion, green part only, chopped, plus extra for garnish

1 clove garlic, chopped

¼ cup cilantro leaves

1½ cups coconut water

juice of ½ lime

pinch of cayenne pepper or ground cumin

full-fat organic yogurt, for garnish

SERVES 2

METHOD

Combine all the ingredients except the yogurt in a blender or food processor until smooth. If the soup is too thick, add more coconut water. Pour into serving bowls and cover with a plate or plastic wrap. Refrigerate for 1 hour. Serve garnished with a dollop of yogurt and some chopped scallion.

SWEET POTATO SOUP

INGREDIENTS

1 tablespoon coconut oil

1 onion, finely chopped

1 teaspoon ground cumin

½ teaspoon ground turmeric

½ teaspoon yellow mustard seeds

pinch of salt

1 cup red lentils, rinsed (optional—if you omit the lentils, add an extra sweet potato)

1 medium sweet potato, peeled and cut into chunks

1 tablespoon tamari or liquid aminos (see Resources, page 205)

freshly ground black pepper, to taste

SERVES 2

METHOD

Heat the coconut oil in a heavy-bottomed saucepan. Add the onion, spices and salt and cook for a few minutes. Add the lentils, sweet potato and ½ cup water and simmer for 30 minutes or until the potato is tender. Add a splash more water if needed, to cover. Season the mixture with the tamari and pepper and purée until smooth and thick. Serve hot.

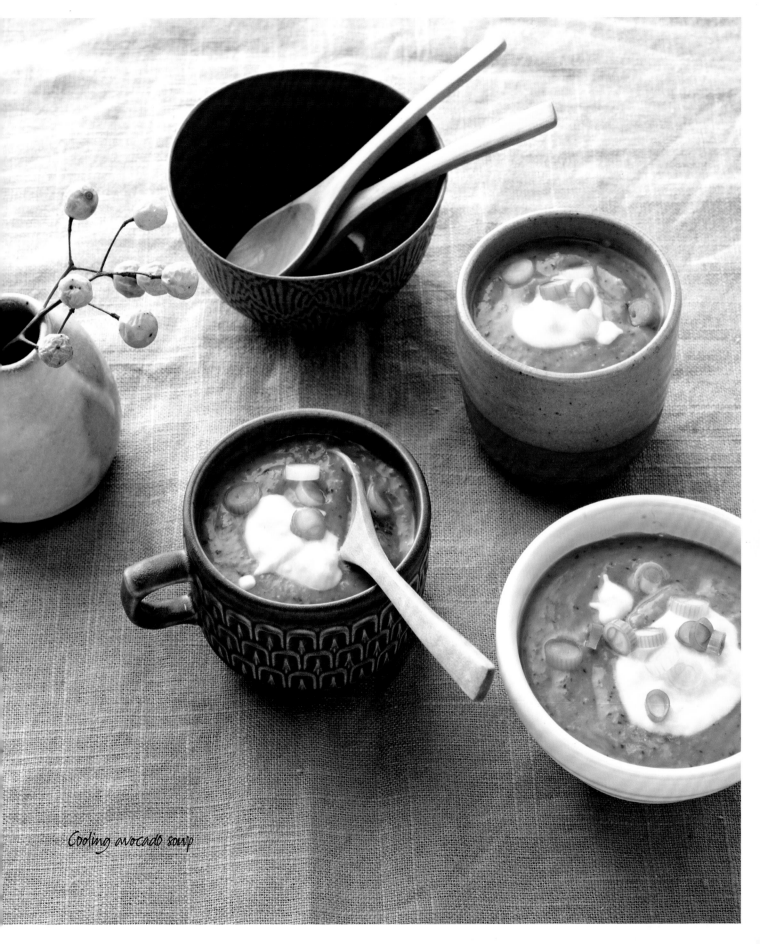

Cooling avocado soup

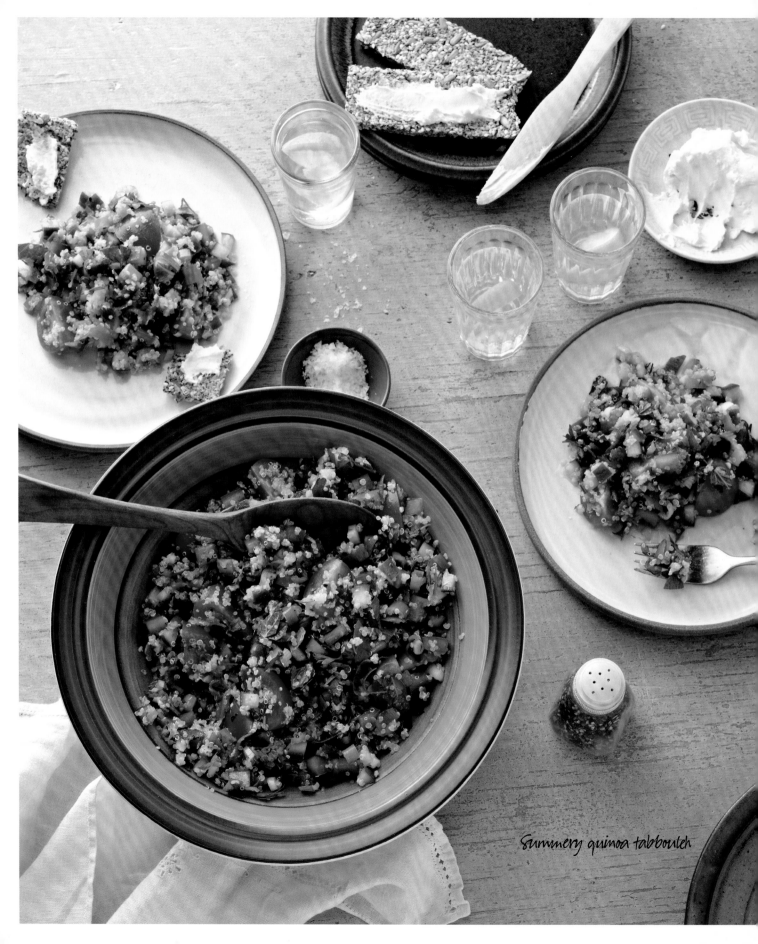

Summery quinoa tabbouleh

SUMMERY QUINOA TABBOULEH

INGREDIENTS

1½ cups cooked quinoa (see page 61)

1 bunch scallions, green parts only, chopped

1 red bell pepper, chopped

1 cup finely diced cucumber

1 cup cherry tomatoes, halved

1 cup chopped flat-leaf parsley

½ cup chopped mint leaves

½ teaspoon ground cumin

½ cup freshly squeezed lemon juice

⅓ cup extra-virgin olive oil

salt and pepper, to taste

SERVES 4–6 AS A SIDE

METHOD

Combine all the ingredients in a large bowl. Allow to sit in the fridge for 1–2 hours before serving.

PEA, HERB AND ALMOND CRUSH

Maria at the Scandi Foodie blog shared this recipe with me.
It's a great vegan toast topper!

INGREDIENTS

14 ounces fresh or frozen peas

1 clove garlic, crushed

1 small bunch chives, roughly chopped

½ cup blanched slivered almonds

salt and freshly ground black pepper, to taste

handful of mixed fresh herbs

zest and juice of 1 lime

1 tablespoon extra-virgin olive oil

MAKES ABOUT 2 CUPS

METHOD

Place the peas, garlic, chives and almonds in a saucepan. Add ¼ cup of water and bring to a boil. Season with salt and pepper and simmer, covered, for 5–10 minutes or until the peas are tender.

Purée the mixed herbs, lime zest and juice and oil to a fine paste in a food processor. Add the herb paste to the peas and mash roughly to mix. Serve on top of fish or pasta or spread on toast. Store any leftovers in an airtight container in the fridge for a few days.

ENDIVE SARDINE BOATS

I love sardines. They're a sustainable fish, super cheap and healthy.
Forget the canned ones—buy fresh and tuck into this recipe for some super nutritious fun.
You can use toast instead of endive, if you wish. This is a great breakfast dish and
makes a fab hors d'oeuvre, too.

INGREDIENTS

6 sardine fillets
½ cup finely chopped flat-leaf parsley
1 long red mild chili, finely chopped
juice and grated zest of ½ lemon
2 tablespoons olive oil
1 Belgian endive
¼ cup homemade Cream Cheese (see page 64)

SERVES 2

METHOD

In a pan cook the sardines over medium heat with a little oil for one minute on each side, until the skin starts to brown a little. Transfer to a small bowl and smash together with the parsley, chili to taste, lemon zest and juice, and oil. Pull apart the endive and top each leaf with a spoonful of cream cheese and some sardine mixture.

NOTE
You can use canned sardines or tuna instead (simply drain the oil or water and skip the cooking step).

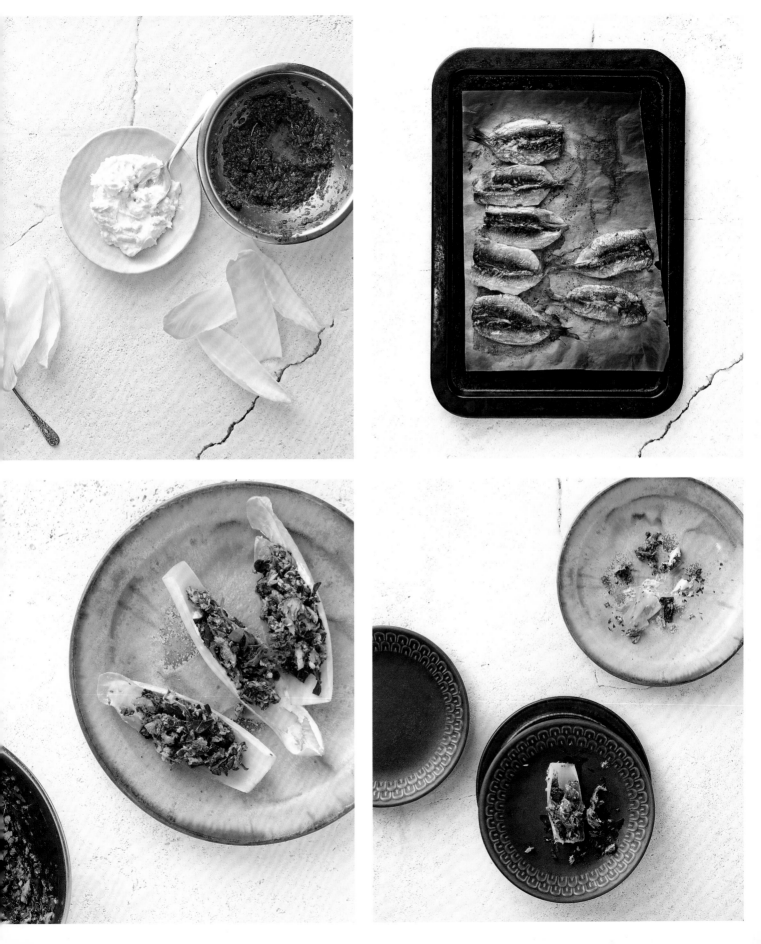

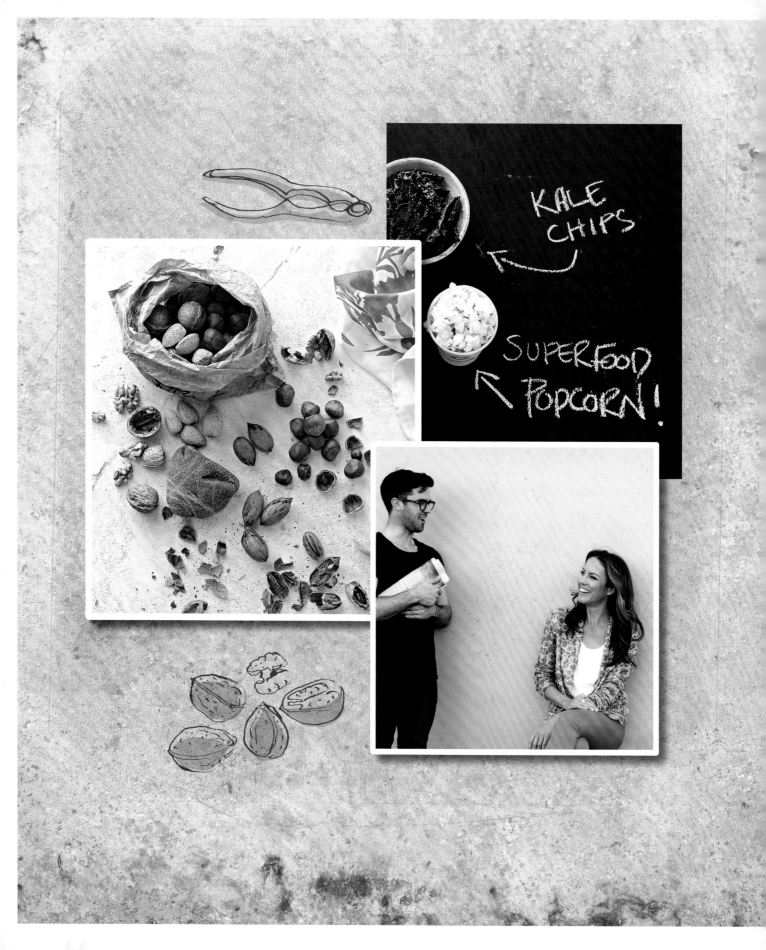

KALE CHIPS

SUPERFOOD POPCORN!

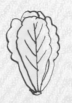

SAVORY SNACKS

For a while during my I Quit Sugar journey, my aim in life was to invent the most nutritious, crunchy, satisfying, portable snack using the least number of ingredients and steps. The recipes in this section are all in the running. Snacks on the savory end of the spectrum, especially those full of good, saturated fats and proteins, are where you want to be heading when you quit sugar. They'll curb cravings and fill you up fast (and provide nutritional oomph), to get you through to your next square meal. Which is the point of a snack, right?

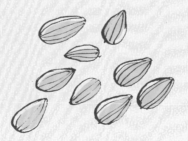

SPROUTED SPICY NUTS

In the first part of this book I showed you how to make Sprouted Nuts and Seeds (see page 59). Here are some ways to jazz them up into a bona fide snack food.

(see page 59)

INGREDIENTS

2 cups walnuts

2 cups almonds

½–1 teaspoon each ground cinnamon, ground coriander and ground cumin

½ teaspoon ground turmeric

MAKES 4 CUPS

METHOD

Toss all the spices through the nuts before drying in the oven.

VARIATIONS:

1. SALT AND VINEGAR ALMONDS

Toss ¼ cup apple cider vinegar and 1 tablespoon salt over 1½ cups of almonds just before you put them in the oven.

2. MEXICAN PUMPKIN SEEDS

Toss the juice of 2–3 limes, 3 teaspoons chili powder and 1 tablespoon salt over 1 cup of pumpkin seeds just before you put them in the oven.

3. TAMARI PUMPKIN SEEDS

After sprouting the pumpkin seeds, toss 1 cup of the seeds into a frying pan over medium-low heat. Add a splash of tamari and stir. The seeds will become a gooey, caramely glob pretty quickly, so remove from the heat almost immediately.

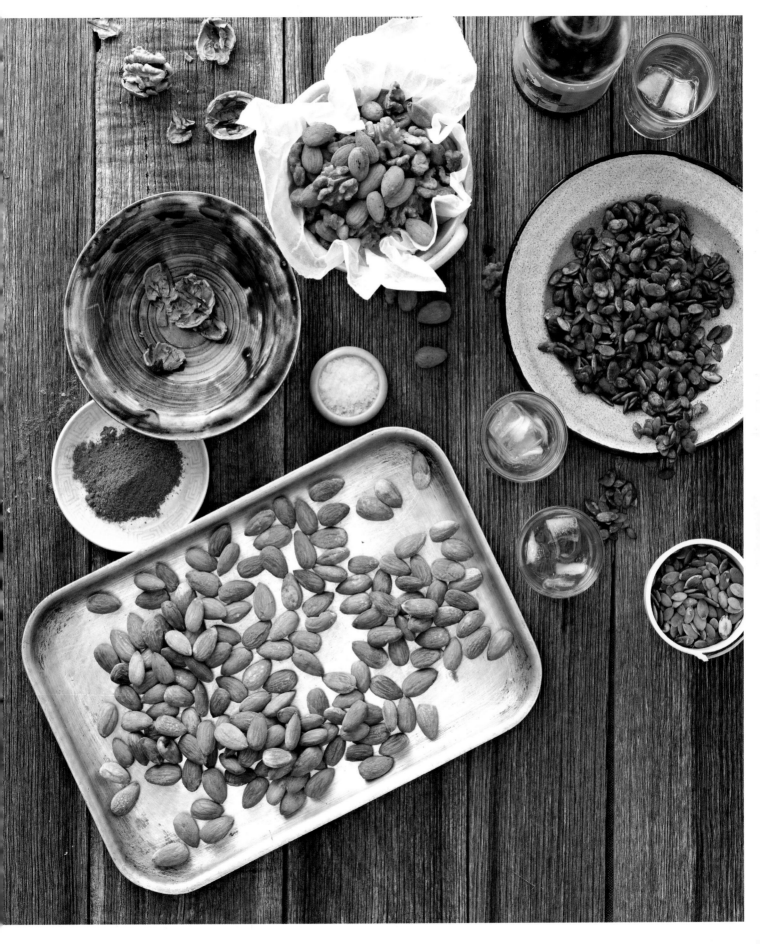

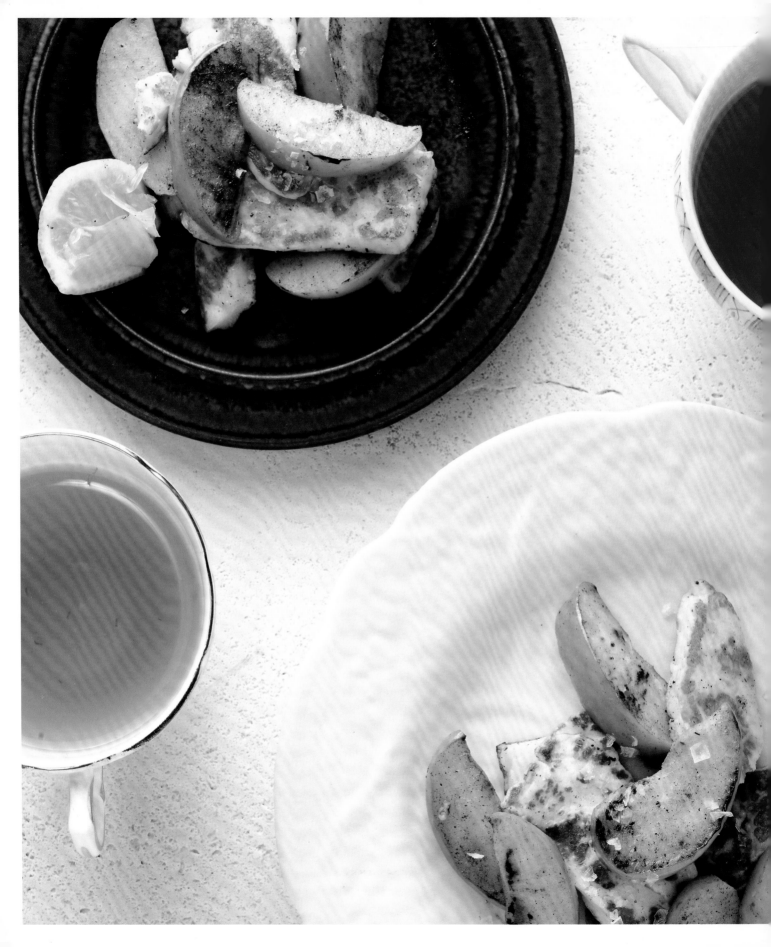

"SALTED CARAMEL" HALOUMI CHEESE AND APPLE

This is a great afternoon snack, or you can serve it with lightly toasted walnuts
as a dessert. Haloumi cheese can now be found in some supermarkets and cheese shops.
It's worth seeking out!

INGREDIENTS

¼ x ¼-in.-thick slices haloumi
1 green apple, cored and cut into ¼-in. wedges
pinch of salt
sprinkle of ground cinnamon (optional)

❄ **BATCH & FREEZE** | **SERVES 2**

METHOD

Place the haloumi and apple slices in a hot non-stick frying pan. Jiggle the pan a little so the fat from the haloumi coats the apple. Cook on both sides for 1–2 minutes, until both the apple and haloumi are a lovely caramel color. Sprinkle with salt and cinnamon (if using) and serve.

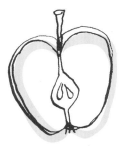

⇨ NO-FUSS SNACK OPTIONS THAT USE THREE INGREDIENTS OR LESS. ⇦

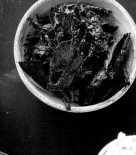

CHICKPEA BOMBS

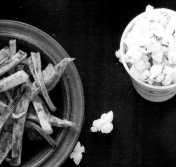

PARSNIP FRIES

CHICKPEA BOMBS

15 oz. can chickpeas (or 1 cup dried chickpeas, soaked overnight and cooked)
1 tablespoon olive oil
1 tablespoon garam masala or ras el hanout

Preheat the oven to 350°F. Drain, rinse, and pat dry the chickpeas, and put in a bowl. Add the olive oil and garam masala and toss to coat. Arrange in a single layer on a baking pan and bake for 45 minutes. Allow to cool. Store leftovers in an airtight container for about a week.

CRISPY BRUSSELS SPROUTS CHIPS

10 Brussels sprouts
1 tablespoon olive oil
¼ teaspoon sea salt

Preheat the oven to 400°F. Cut off the bottom tip of each sprout and peel off the leaves. Toss the leaves with the oil (coat well) and lay in one layer on a baking pan. Sprinkle with the salt and bake 8–10 minutes, until the leaves are lightly browned and crisp. Eat them right away (they go soggy after a few hours).

NOTE

This is a great way to use up the outer leaves of your sprouts. I prefer to keep the "hearts" for another use and only use the leaves for these chips.

TOASTY WATER CHESTNUTS

can water chestnuts, drained
coconut, macadamia or sesame oil

Heat in a pan with a little oil until golden. Serve.

> **NOTE**
> Canned water chestnuts are inexpensive and available in the Asian food section of most supermarkets. Cook them in your favorite oil.

DAIKON CHIPS

2 large daikon
2 tablespoons coconut oil, melted (or sesame or olive oil)
salt and chopped rosemary, to taste

Preheat the oven to 400°F and line a baking pan with parchment paper. Cut the daikon into 5 mm slices, using a sharp knife or mandoline. Toss all the ingredients in a bowl to coat the daikon, then arrange on the pan and bake for 20 minutes. Turn off the heat and leave the daikon to sit in the oven for 10 minutes to crisp up. Serve immediately.

> **NOTE**
> Daikon are large, long white radishes found in Asian food stores. They're often grated over salads in Japanese restaurants. Turnips are a good substitute if you can't find any.

KALE CHIPS

1 bunch kale or cavolo nero (2¾ cup), stalks removed
1 tablespoon olive oil
pinch of salt

Preheat the oven to 400°F. Tear the kale roughly into 1½ in. squares. Toss in the oil and salt, then lay on a baking pan and cook for 5–10 minutes until crisp. Can be eaten either hot or cold.

> **NOTE**
> Never eat kale stalks—they are too hard to digest. The easiest way to remove the stalks is to grab the stalk end and then run your fingers down it, shearing the leaf off (see page 126).

QUICK SNACKS

SUPERFOOD POPCORN

small handful of popping corn
knob of butter or coconut oil
1 tablespoon dulse flakes

To make in the microwave, put the popping corn and butter in a brown paper bag and roll down the top to close. Microwave on high for 2 minutes. Add the dulse flakes to the bag and shake. Serve.

To make on the stove, melt the butter in a frying pan. Add the popping corn and cover until the popping slows. Transfer to a serving bowl and toss through the dulse flakes. Serve.

> **VARIATION**
> For a cheesy flavor, instead of the dulse flakes use 1 tablespoon nutritional yeast and 1 tablespoon tamari or liquid aminos. (See Resources, page 205).

PARSNIP FRIES

INGREDIENTS

3 tablespoons chunky unsalted unsweetened peanut butter or almond butter (see page 64 for recipe)

1 tablespoon olive oil

salt, to taste

3 parsnips or 1 celery root, peeled and cut into thin sticks

SERVES 1 OR 2

METHOD

Preheat the oven to 400°F and line a baking pan with parchment paper. Mix the nut butter, oil and salt. Add the parsnips and toss with your hands to coat. Arrange on the baking pan and bake for about 45 minutes, until crisp. Serve immediately.

POTATO SKINS

Sally Fallon is a hero of mine, and her *Nourishing Traditions* cookbook is permanently open on my kitchen counter. She happily shared this recipe with me recently. Sally cooks like your grandmother used to, with full nutritional zing as the focus.

INGREDIENTS

4 large baking potatoes

3 tablespoons butter, melted

1 cup grated cheese (Cheddar or Monterey Jack)

1 bunch scallions, green parts only, finely chopped, to serve (optional)

sour cream, guacamole, crispy bacon bits, to serve (optional)

SERVES 1 OR 2

METHOD

Preheat the oven to 350°F. Wash and dry the potatoes, then brush with melted butter. Bake until soft. Leave the oven on. Split the potatoes lengthwise and scoop out the flesh (use it for mashed potato, or Foolproof Fennel Soup on page 123). Brush the potato skins inside and out with melted butter and bake for about 30 minutes or until crisp. Serve with the cheese sprinkled on the top and, if desired, scallions, sour cream and other accompaniments.

CHEESY BISCUITS

These use coconut flour, so they are chewy and dense (see page 69).
Two of these and you'll be stuffed like a Thanksgiving turkey for hours.

INGREDIENTS

½ cup almond meal, hempseed meal or other nut meal

3 eggs

4 tablespoons butter, melted

a good grind or two of salt

generous shake of chili flakes or paprika

2 cups grated Cheddar cheese

½–¾ cup coconut flour, sifted

chopped cherry tomatoes and basil leaves, to serve

❊ BATCH & FREEZE ❘ MAKES 16

METHOD

Preheat the oven to 400°F and line a baking pan with parchment paper. Blend the almond meal, eggs, butter, salt, chili flakes and cheese. Add ½ cup of the coconut flour and knead the dough until moist and the consistency of Play-Doh. Add a little more flour if necessary. If the dough seems too dry, add another egg, extra melted butter or a little coconut water. Form the dough into walnut-sized balls and put on the pan. Flatten each ball until ½ in. thick (or less if you want thin crackers). Bake for 15 minutes, until golden and crisp, turning once. Serve with chopped cherry tomatoes and basil leaves.

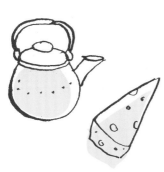

MEAL-IN-A-CRACKER

Serve these crackers with dips, mashed avocado or homemade Cream Cheese
(see page 64), or keep some at work for an afternoon snack fix.

INGREDIENTS

½ cup chia seeds

½ cup sunflower seeds

½ cup sesame seeds

½ cup almond meal, hempseed meal
or other nut meal

2 cloves garlic, crushed

2 teaspoons freshly chopped herbs (I like sage for these)

1 teaspoon dulse flakes (optional)

¼ teaspoon salt

MAKES 20

METHOD

Preheat the oven to 325°F and line a baking pan
with parchment paper. Combine the seeds and
almond meal in a bowl. In a separate bowl, whisk
the remaining ingredients with 1 cup water. Pour
the liquid mixture onto the seed mixture and stir
until thick and combined. Spread the mixture on
the pan, pressing down using the back of a spoon,
until it is ¼ in. thick. Bake for 30 minutes. Remove
from the oven, cut into 20 crackers using a knife,
flip them over and bake for another 25 minutes.
Allow to cool completely on the pan. Store in a
sealed container for two weeks.

I hike a lot. When I do, I take just a hat, map and a key, a cucumber and some of these crackin' crackers.

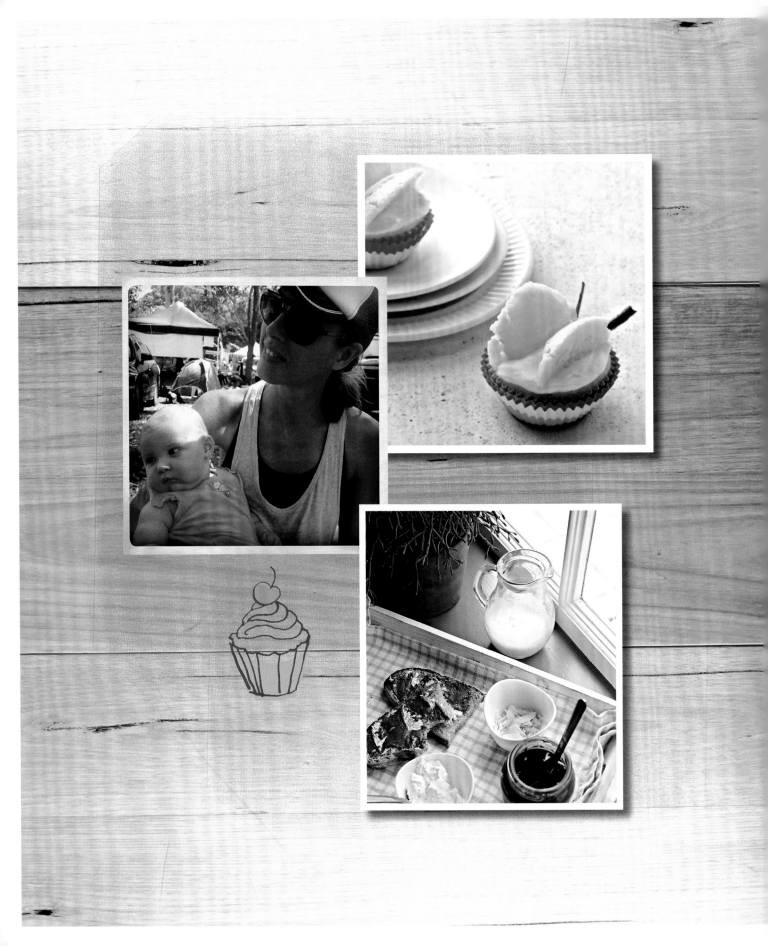

SUGAR-FREE KIDS

⇨ SOME SERIOUSLY CONVINCING INDULGENCES
FOR THE LITTLE ONES. ⇦

One of the questions I get asked most is, "How in the world do I get my kids to go sugar free?" It's a good, fair question because kids are almost force-fed the stuff from every angle and denying them access can seem cruel. I mean, what to do at kids' parties? What to pack in their lunchboxes that won't leave them the laughingstock on the playground? And how to navigate the minefield of competing messages that are geared at confused parents?

What to do? Well, I think these recipes are a healthy start.

AVOCADO AND COCONUT POPSICLES

INGREDIENTS

1 large ripe avocado

1 cup coconut cream (see Note, page 167)

juice of 1 lime

3 tablespoons coconut water

1 tablespoon brown rice syrup

1 teaspoon chia seeds (preferably white ones)

¼ teaspoon salt

MAKES 6–8

METHOD

Blend all the ingredients in a food processor or use an immersion blender. Beat to a creamy liquid. Spoon the mixture into ice-cream molds, then insert the sticks. Freeze for at least 4 hours.

VARIATION

You can also make these with the flesh of a baby coconut rather than avocado, using an additional 3 tablespoons of coconut water.

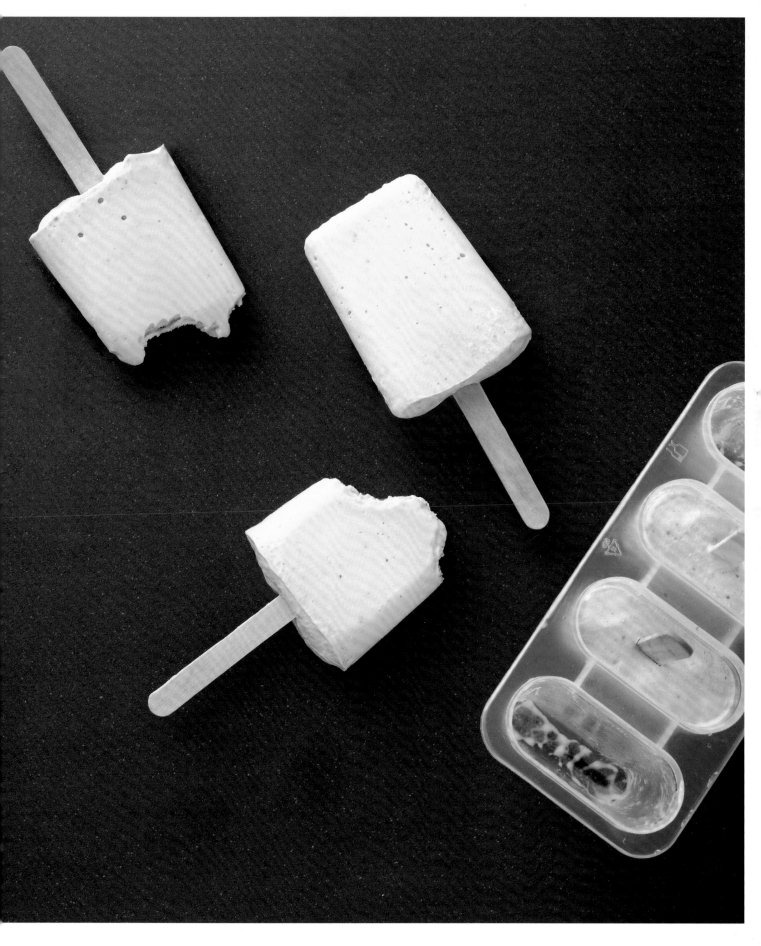

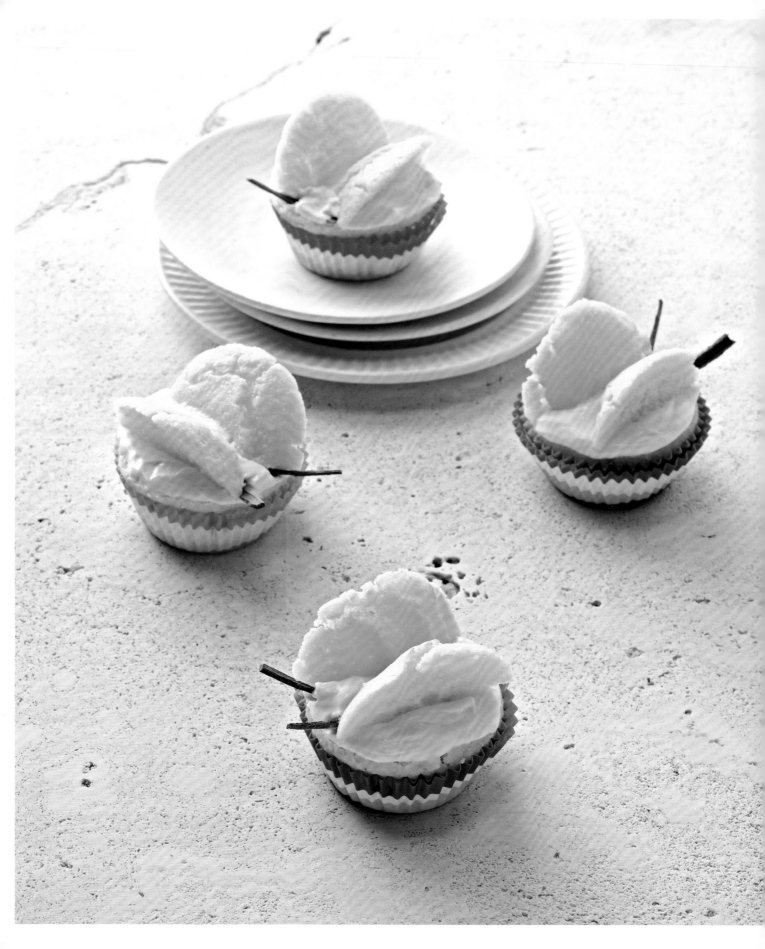

BUTTERFLY CUPCAKES

My mum used to make these for us as kids. A little bit of novelty can go a long way to making a basic recipe buzz! Of course, you can make them as straightforward cupcakes, too.

INGREDIENTS

1 cup milk

1 tablespoon lemon juice or apple cider vinegar

2 large eggs

3 tablespoons powdered stevia

1¼ cups self-rising flour, sifted

¼ cup almond meal

2 teaspoons baking powder

1 teaspoon vanilla powder

7 tablespoons unsalted butter, softened

2 tablespoons sour cream or yogurt

CREAM CHEESE ICING

1½ cups homemade Cream Cheese (see page 64)

3 tablespoons powdered stevia

1 teaspoon natural vanilla extract

3 tablespoons heavy cream

MAKES 12

NOTE
Use cinnamon-stick shards or toothpicks for the butterfly antennae.

METHOD

Preheat the oven to 350°F and line a 12-cup muffin pan with cupcake papers. Combine the milk and lemon juice and let sit for 5 minutes. Blend the eggs and stevia for 5 minutes or until very thick and creamy. Add the flour, almond meal, baking powder, vanilla powder, butter and sour cream. Pour in the milk mixture and beat lightly until well combined. Spoon into the cupcake papers and bake for 12–15 minutes, until firm and a skewer inserted comes out clean. Remove from the oven and allow to cool on wire racks.

To make the icing, blend the cream cheese, stevia and vanilla extract with an immersion blender. Add 1 tablespoon of cream at a time until you reach a smooth, creamy consistency. Using a bread knife, cut off the top of each cupcake (the part that extends over the edge of the paper), then cut each cupcake top in half. Spread a layer of icing over each cupcake, then arrange the 2 top pieces to resemble butterfly wings.

"WHAT DO I FEED THE KIDS?"

OVER THE PAST TWO YEARS OF VOICING MY SUGAR-FREE MESSAGE
I'VE COLLATED SOME TIPS AND SOME GREAT LUNCHBOX IDEAS
FROM EXPERTS, FRIENDS AND COMMENTERS ON MY BLOG.

LEAD BY EXAMPLE

Don't keep sugar in the house. At all. Avoid talking about it, too. The more that the sugar-free experience is normalized, the more kids will slip into line.

GET THE KIDS INVOLVED

Take them shopping and have them help you find the "good" sugar-free yogurt, the cereal with no sugar, and have them find the best stuff to eat in the school cafeteria and when out at restaurants. The more they own the process, the less friction.

BREAKFAST CEREALS

The best—and possibly only—options are Post Shredded Wheat Original, Quaker Puffed Rice, or Kashi 7 Whole Grain Cereal Puffs. Everything else is laden with sugar, apart from a few fruit-free granola options out there (but check the nutritional label to make sure honey hasn't been added). Look for any cereal with less than 2g of sugar per serving. Trick up these options with a sprinkle of my Coco-Nutty Granola (see page 76).

KEEP FLAVORS SIMPLE

A bunch of regular readers of my blog recommend using the IQS experience to get kids back to the simple—as in, one or two—flavors they like.

TREAT WITH OTHER THINGS

My best mate Ragni, who has three kids under seven, says: "The rod many parents make for themselves is to reward with food . . . I try really hard not to do this and to reward them with fun experiences—doing a puzzle, going to the beach, making some pasta together!"

AT PARTIES

Oh, dear. This is hard. My only advice—as gleaned from many, many moms and dads—is not to worry about parties. Let them do their thing. And hopefully two things will happen. One, the practices instilled at home will mean your kids will be more focused on playing games than hovering around the sprinkle cookies. Two, after a few mouthfuls of hideous orange soda they'll feel sufficiently ill and work out they'd really rather some water instead.

SOME SIMPLE LUNCHBOX IDEAS

- A small container of plain yogurt with frozen berries (which will keep it cool until mid-morning).

- Cheese and crackers.

- A Chewy Squash and Coconut Muffin (see page 80) with some homemade Cream Cheese (see page 64).

- A zip-lock bag of Coco-Nutty Granola (see page 76).

- I like the "Fish and Chips" idea David Gillespie shared with me a while back—a small can of tuna with a small bag of potato chips.

- Celery sticks lined with nut butter (see page 64). Nicole on my blog adds mung beans on top and calls it a "celery log boat" (I used to call it "ants on a log" as a kid).

- A frozen carton of coconut water (which will go nice and slushy by lunchtime).

- Lauren says, "I bake a sweet potato, remove the skin, then add avocado, cinnamon, coconut, even cacao powder. I give it a quick spin in the food processor and my one-and-a-half-year old goes crazy for it."

- Sweet coconut chips: unsweetened coconut flakes lightly toasted with cinnamon (great for after school, too).

- Apple sandwiches. I make these for myself! Almond butter (see page 64) spread between apple slices, or a chunk of cheese between two slices of apple.

- Blog reader Nat carries hard-boiled eggs in her bag at all times for her younger kids.

- Wrap slices of ham around a pickle, cucumber or avocado.

- Seaweed snacks. You can find these little packets in Asian grocers—great for a "something in a packet" fix.

- Kimberly suggests guacamole (just mash avocado and lime juice) and vegetable sticks. She gets her sons to mash the guacamole.

- Superfood Popcorn (see recipe on page 151). My mom used to do this when I was a kid and microwaves were first invented.

- Sugar snap peas.

- A great afternoon snack idea: corn tortillas with hot melted Cheddar cheese. Place on a baking pan and stick them under the broiler until they're warm and the cheese is melted and bubbly.

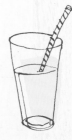

ZEST-AND-POPPY COOKIES

INGREDIENTS

2 tablespoons grapeseed oil

1½ tablespoons granulated stevia

1 tablespoon vanilla powder

1 tablespoon grated lemon zest

1¾ cups almond meal

pinch of salt

1 tablespoon poppy seeds

1 egg white, lightly beaten

MAKES 12–16

METHOD

Preheat the oven to 350°F. In a large bowl, combine the oil, stevia, vanilla powder and lemon zest. Add the almond meal, salt and poppy seeds and work with your fingers for a good 5 minutes to release the oil in the meal and form a good dough. Roll out the dough to about ½ to ¾ in. thick, then cut into shapes using a cookie cutter. Brush with the egg white to give the cookies a pretty gloss. Bake for 6–8 minutes, until light golden brown around the edges.

TIPS

- Use a bunny-shaped cutter to make Easter cookies.
- If you can't be bothered with cookie cutters, roll the dough into balls and squish them flat instead.

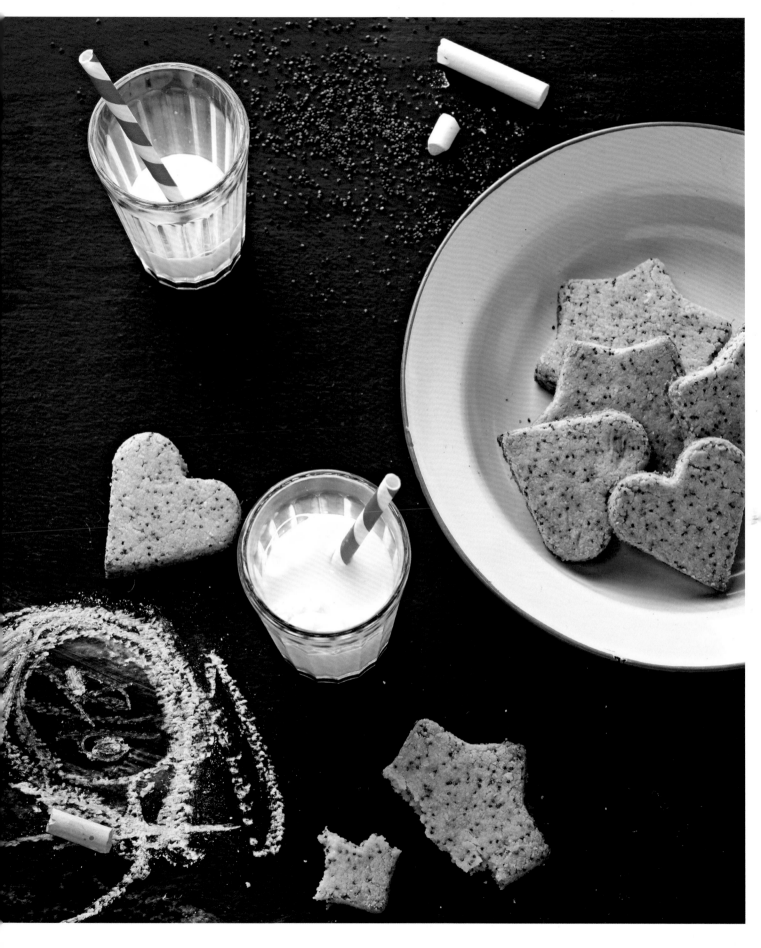

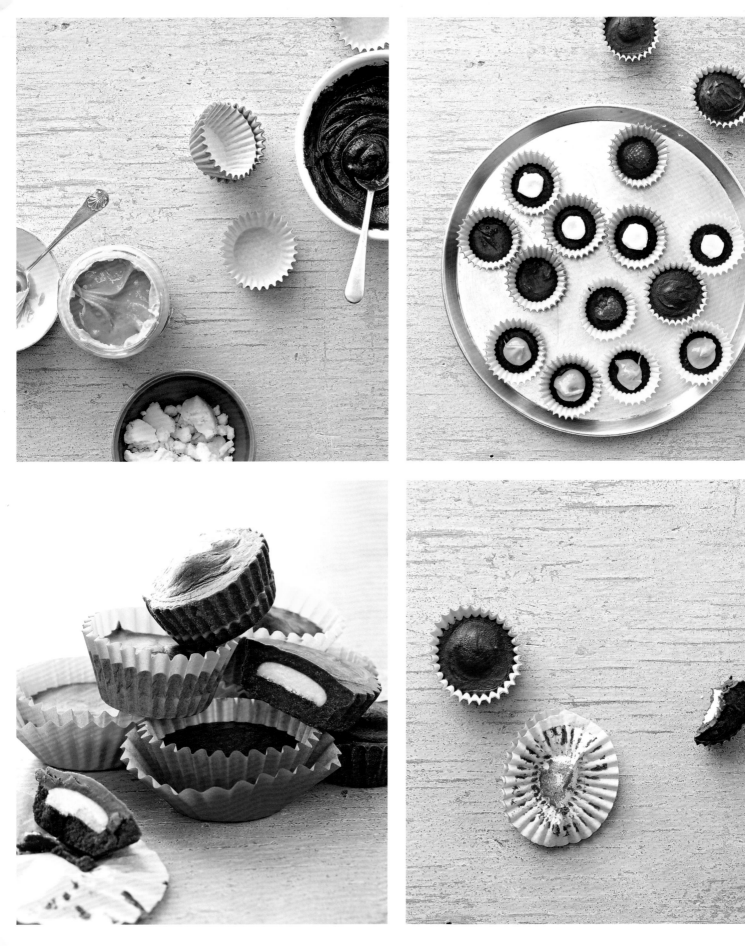

CHOCOLATE NUT BUTTER CUPS

You know those junky peanut butter cups you can buy? Well, these are same-same-but-way-better. The coconut cream in this recipe makes the "chocolate" smoother. Interestingly, I find the more coconut cream you use, the harder the chocolate texture.

INGREDIENTS

½ cup coconut oil, melted
½ cup raw cacao powder
1 tablespoon brown rice syrup
2 tablespoons coconut cream
¼ cup peanut, macadamia or almond butter
large pinch of sea salt

MAKES ABOUT 20–25

NOTE

If coconut cream, which can be found at some supermarkets and Asian food stores, is unavailable, you can substitute coconut milk. To thicken it, add 1 tablespoon of arrowroot for each cup of coconut milk.

METHOD

Arrange small paper candy cups on a baking pan. In a small bowl, combine the coconut oil and cacao powder until smooth, then stir in the syrup and coconut cream. Pour a thin layer into the bottom of the candy cups. Freeze for 5 minutes, then remove from the freezer and spoon ⅓ teaspoon of the nut butter into each one. Pour the remaining cacao mixture on top and scatter sea salt over. Refrigerate for 30 minutes until set (or, if you're short of time, freeze them). Eat straight from the fridge—these will melt at room temperature.

TRY THESE DELICIOUS VARIATIONS:

1. **COCONUT BUTTER CUPS**
   Make a coconut version by using a small ball of Coconut Butter (see page 182) instead of the nut butter.

2. **PEPPERMINT PATTIES**
   Make peppermint patties by adding a few drops of peppermint oil (to taste) to small balls of Coconut Butter (see page 182) instead of the nut butter.

3. **BERRY CUPS**
   Make a berry version by placing a frozen raspberry in the middle instead of the nut butter.

SUGAR-FREE "NUTELLA"

The processed version of this spread is a dire sugar explosion.
This one, though, will fool even the most skeptical child.

INGREDIENTS

1 cup hazelnuts
½ cup coconut milk
⅓ cup brown rice syrup
1 tablespoon macadamia oil (or coconut oil)
¼ cup raw cacao powder
1 tablespoon vanilla powder

MAKES ABOUT 1 CUP

METHOD

Preheat the oven to 350°F. Bake the hazelnuts on a baking pan for 8–10 minutes, until browned. Rub off most of the skins, as they can be bitter (you don't have to be too precise). Grind the nuts in a food processor until smooth. Add the remaining ingredients and process until well mixed. Add extra coconut milk if you want more of a "sauce" consistency. Store in the fridge for several weeks.

FLUFFY CARROT MOUSSE

INGREDIENTS

coconut oil or butter for greasing
5–6 cups chopped carrots
¼ cup almond meal
3 eggs
2 tablespoons brown rice syrup
½ teaspoon ground nutmeg
½ teaspoon ground cinnamon
1 tablespoon grated orange zest

SERVES 4

METHOD

Preheat the oven to 350°F and lightly grease a small baking dish. Steam the carrots for 15–20 minutes, until soft. Transfer to a blender and blend with the remaining ingredients until smooth. Pour the mixture into the baking dish and bake for 1 hour until browned around the edges and done in the center. Serve warm straight from the oven or allow to cool, then refrigerate overnight and serve cold.

VARIATION
Whip up a batch and pour into individual ovenproof cups or ramekins for an after-school snack.

Sugar-free "nutella" on a bit of toast.
I take mine on rice thins.

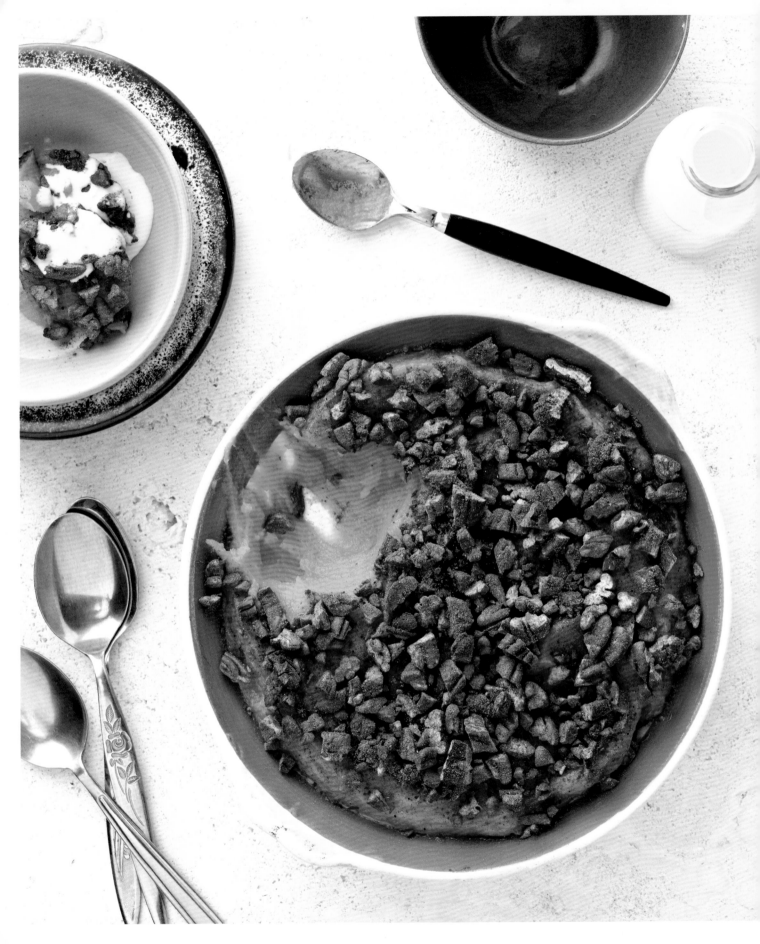

SWEET POTATO CASSEROLE

As well as a dessert, this is a great side dish for "special-ish" occasions or an easy Sunday night no-fuss meal.

INGREDIENTS

coconut oil or butter for greasing
3 cups Sweet Potato Purée (see Variation, page 58)
3 tablespoons homemade Almond Milk (see page 65)
1 tablespoon brown rice syrup
1 teaspoon vanilla powder
pinch of salt
½ cup chopped pecans, preferably sprouted (see page 59)
1 teaspoon ground cinnamon
½ teaspoon ground ginger
½ teaspoon ground allspice

SERVES 4–6

METHOD

Preheat the oven to 350°F and lightly grease a small baking dish. Combine the sweet potato, almond milk, syrup, vanilla powder and salt and pour into the baking dish. Toss the remaining ingredients in a small bowl, then sprinkle evenly on top of the sweet potato mixture. Bake for 30 minutes. Serve immediately, with cream (whipped, if desired) if having for dessert.

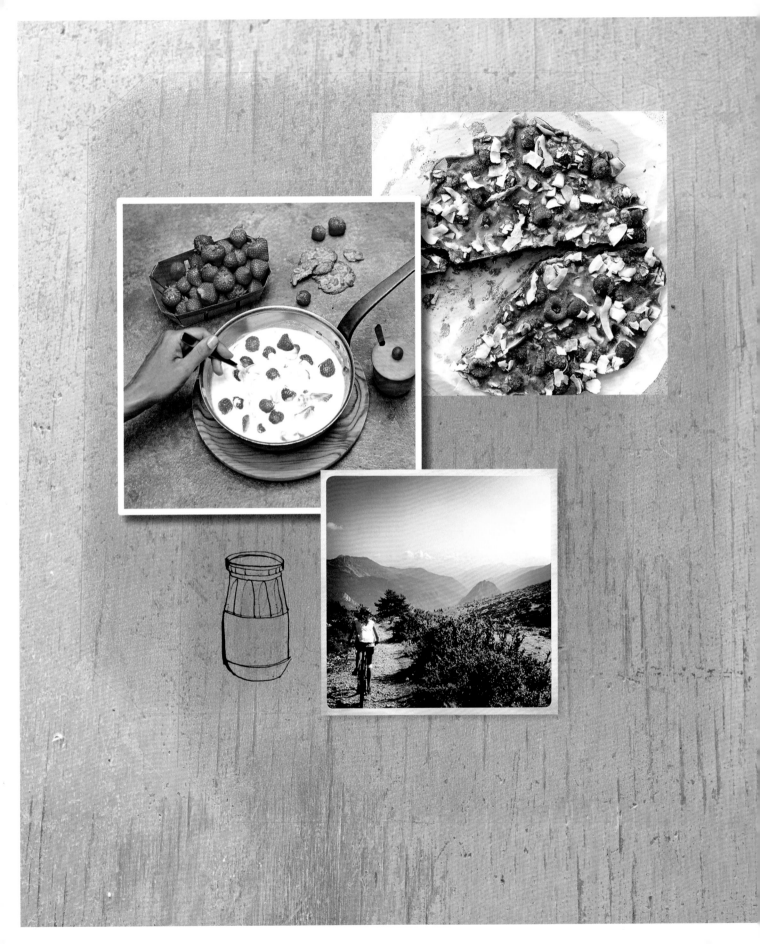

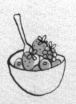

SWEET TREATS

⇨ SWEET *AND* SUGAR-FREE. IN FACT, ALL THESE SIMPLE SNACKS ARE GOOD ENOUGH TO EAT FOR BREAKFAST ⇦

The recipes I've assembled here are the kinds of things you can make in an instant when a craving hits.They look and taste like explosive indulgences, but on closer inspection contain highly nutritious ingredients—coconut, nuts, cream, low-fructose fruit and raw cacao. Many of the recipes are also left uncooked, leaving the crucial enzymes intact. That said, they are designed to take the place of your sweet treats of yore, so they're still occasional indulgences, not meal substitutes, okay?

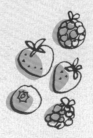

ALMOND BUTTER BARK

This is one of my favorite treats. Hand it out to fans of salted caramel and see
if it doesn't make them smile in blissful surprise.

INGREDIENTS

⅓ cup coconut oil, melted

¼ cup almond butter, slightly warmed or melted

2 tablespoons unsweetened coconut flakes

2 teaspoons brown rice syrup

pinch of rock salt, ground

handful of cacao nibs or dark (85% cacao) chocolate shavings

MAKES 12–15 SHARDS

METHOD

Line a baking pan with baking paper. Combine the oil, almond butter, coconut flakes and syrup in a bowl. Spread on the pan and sprinkle with salt and cacao nibs. Freeze for about 20 minutes, then snap into shards. Store in an airtight container in the fridge (the shards will melt if left out at room temperature).

VARIATION

If you don't have any almond butter, make some by combining 5 tablespoons softened butter and ⅓ cup almond meal, hempseed meal or other nut meal.

CANDIED PECANS

INGREDIENTS

butter for greasing

3 egg whites

pinch of salt

⅓ cup brown rice syrup

1 tablespoon vanilla powder

4 cups pecans

MAKES 4 CUPS

METHOD

Preheat the oven to 175°F and grease 2 baking pans with butter. In a clean, dry bowl, beat the egg whites with the salt. Slowly beat in the syrup and vanilla powder, then fold in the pecans until they are well coated. Spread on the pans and place in the oven for several hours until the egg-white coating hardens. Store in an airtight container in the fridge for 2 weeks.

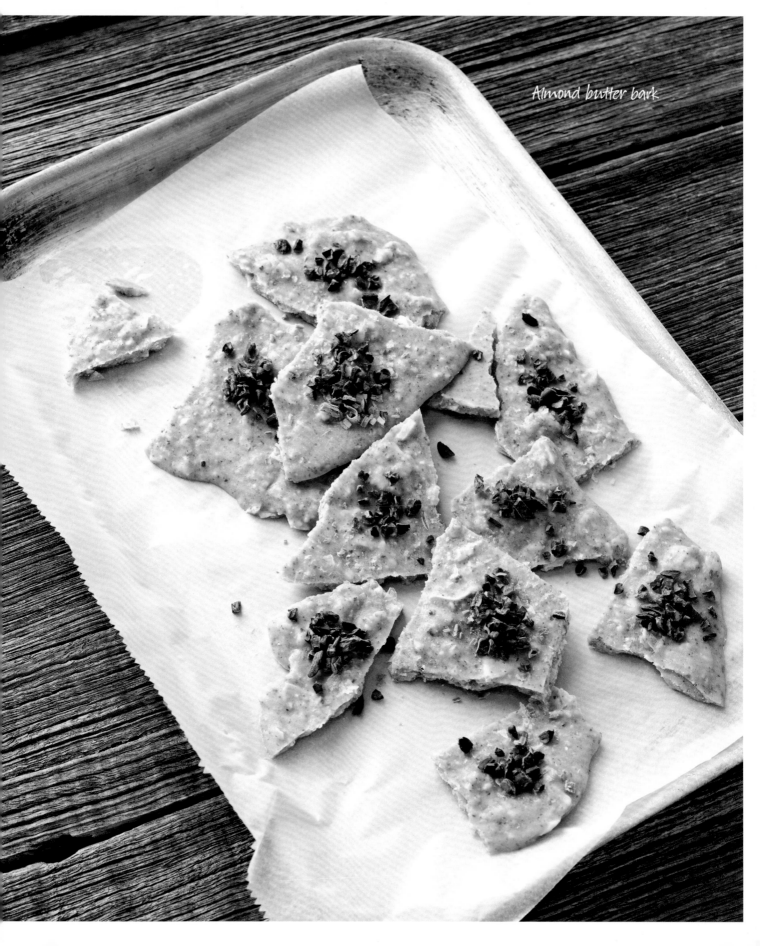

GRAPEFRUTTI-TUTTI CAKE

INGREDIENTS

coconut oil or butter for greasing

zest and juice of 1 grapefruit (you need ⅓ cup juice)

⅓ cup brown rice syrup

½ cup homemade Almond Milk (see page 65)
or other milk

3 large eggs, lightly beaten

½ cup extra-virgin olive oil (or ⅓ cup olive oil plus ⅓ cup
melted coconut oil)

1 cup millet flour, brown rice flour or quinoa flour
(or a combination of all three)

¼ cup coconut flour

¼ cup arrowroot

1½ teaspoons baking powder

¼ teaspoon baking soda

¼ teaspoon salt

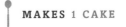 **MAKES** 1 **CAKE**

METHOD

Preheat the oven to 350°F. Grease and line a 9-in. square pan with baking paper. Alternatively grease a Bundt pan. Stir the grapefruit zest into the syrup and set aside to steep. Mix the grapefruit juice with the milk and add to the zest-infused syrup, whisking. Stir the eggs and oil into the zest and syrup mixture.

Sift the remaining ingredients. Add this to the zest and syrup mixture, gradually stirring until the lumps disappear and the batter thickens. Pour the batter into the pan and bake for 45 minutes. Remove from the oven and allow to cool on a rack.

CHEWY QUINOA MACAROONS

INGREDIENTS

3 large or 4 medium egg whites

⅓ cup brown rice syrup

1½ cups unsweetened shredded coconut

1 cup cooked quinoa (see page 61)

pinch of salt

MAKES ABOUT 12

METHOD

Whisk the egg whites and syrup. Stir in the coconut, quinoa and salt and place in the fridge for 1 hour. Preheat the oven to 325°F and line a baking pan with baking paper. Scoop the quinoa mixture into "blobs" and arrange on the pan. Use your fingers to mold the blobs into small domes. Bake for 15 minutes, until golden brown. Allow to cool.

FUDGY PROTEIN BITES

INGREDIENTS

1½ cups basic raw chocolate

¾ cup vanilla protein powder

½ cup chia seeds

⅓ cup maca powder, optional (if not using maca powder, add a little extra protein powder)

MAKES 15–30

METHOD

Combine all of the ingredients and pour immediately into silicon molds or cupcake papers (mini or standard) and place in the fridge or freezer to harden.

NOTE

To make basic raw chocolate: Blend 1½ cups coconut oil, ½ cup raw cacao powder, 2 tablespoons brown rice syrup and 2 pinches of sea salt until smooth. Pour into molds or onto a baking paper–lined plate and refrigerate or freeze.

SWEET POTATO TRUFFLE BALLS

INGREDIENTS

1 cup Sweet Potato Purée (see Variation, page 58)

3 tablespoons coconut oil, melted

2 tablespoons coconut cream (see Note, page 167)

1 tablespoon coconut flour

1 teaspoon granulated stevia or 1–2 teaspoons brown rice syrup

pinch of salt

handful of unsweetened shredded coconut (toasted if you like)

MAKES ABOUT 16

METHOD

Combine all the ingredients except the shredded coconut, stirring well. Cover and refrigerate for at least 1 hour. Scoop out teaspoonfuls and roll into balls, then roll in the coconut. Store in the fridge in an airtight container for a week.

SPIRULINA AND SESAME BALLS

INGREDIENTS

1 cup nuts (almonds or brazil nuts are best), preferably sprouted (see page 59)

½ cup almond butter

½ cup tahini

½ cup almond meal

¼ cup sesame seeds, plus extra for coating

1 tablespoon spirulina powder

1 teaspoon granulated stevia

MAKES ABOUT 12

METHOD

Line a baking pan with baking paper. Roughly chop the nuts in a food processor. Combine all the ingredients in a bowl, mixing until smooth. Add extra almond meal if the mixture feels a bit wet, or extra tahini if it feels a bit dry. Grab small handfuls and roll into balls, then roll in the extra sesame seeds to coat. Place on the pan and refrigerate for 1 hour. The balls will keep for several weeks in an airtight container in the fridge.

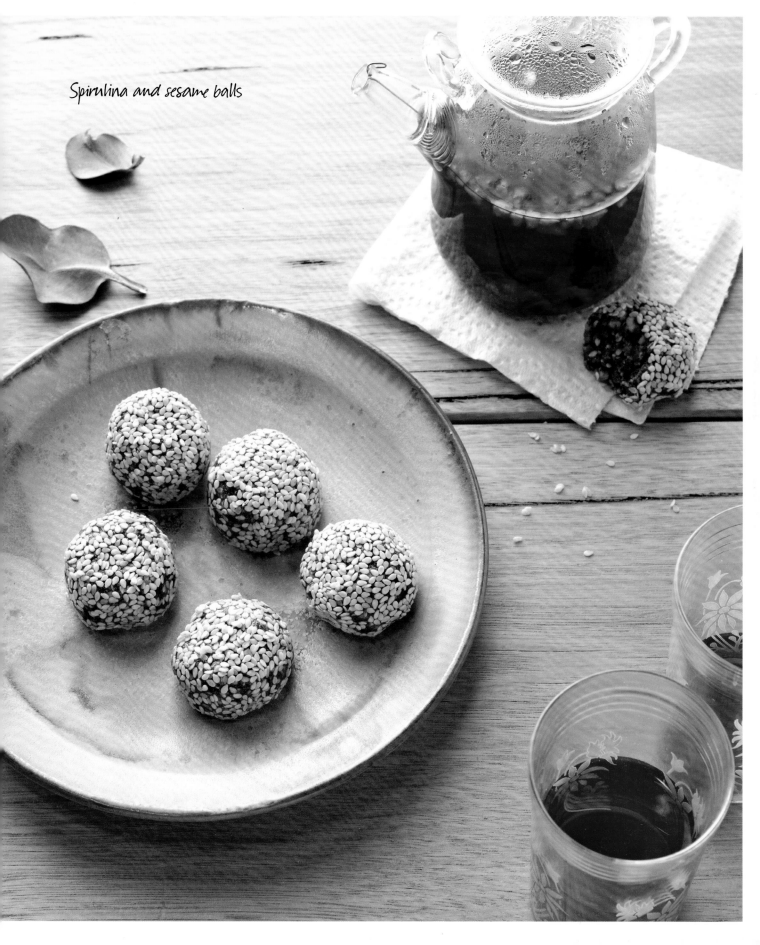

Spirulina and sesame balls

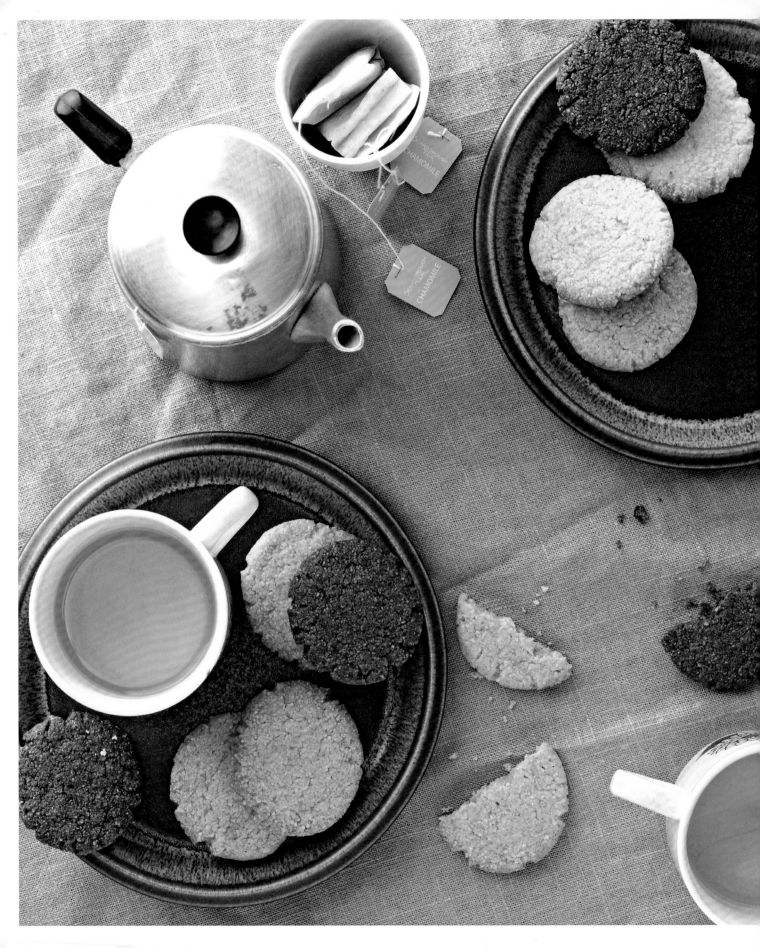

SIMPLY SWEET COOKIES

INGREDIENTS

2½ cups almond meal

½ teaspoon baking soda

½ teaspoon sea salt

8 tablespoons butter, softened

⅓ cup powdered stevia

1 teaspoon vanilla powder

MAKES ABOUT 30

METHOD

Preheat the oven to 350°F and line a baking pan with baking paper. Pulse the almond meal, baking soda and salt briefly in a food processor. Add the butter, stevia and vanilla powder and blend a little more. Spoon heaped tablespoons of the mixture onto the baking pan and press down with your hand to flatten. Bake for about 8 minutes, until golden. Allow to cool on wire racks.

THREE LOVELY VARIATIONS:

1. **MOCHA CHIP COOKIES**
   Add ½ cup sugar-free chocolate chopped into small chunks (or ½ cup cacao nibs), 3 tablespoons raw cacao powder and 1½ tablespoons ground coffee to the mixture.

2. **SOPHISTICATED LAVENDER SNAPS**
   Add 2 teaspoons finely chopped dried lavender and 1 tablespoon finely grated orange zest and blend for an extra 10 seconds.

3. **GINGERBREAD CHEWS**
   Add 1 tablespoon ground ginger, 1 teaspoon ground nutmeg, 1 teaspoon ground cinnamon and 1 tablespoon finely grated orange zest, and blend for an extra 10 seconds.

⇨ BY NOW YOU ARE PROBABLY VERY AWARE THAT I ADVOCATE GETTING WELL SETTLED ON THE COCONUT TRAIN WHEN QUITTING SUGAR. HERE ARE SOME FUN WAYS TO DO SO. ⇦

COCONUT BUTTER

This is the cheapest, easiest, most nutritious and damn tastiest thing in this book. The processing takes some patience with a regular food processor or blender, but be sure not to give up before the mixture turns runny—it simply won't taste the same. Also, always use a whole package of coconut: the recipe doesn't work with small quantities because the lack of volume means it won't "take" to the blender.

INGREDIENTS
1 packet unsweetened shredded coconut (bigger is better)

MAKES 1 JAR

TIP
Pour the coconut butter into paper candy cups or molds or into an ice-cube tray, and keep in the fridge to use as a white chocolate truffle-ish indulgence.

METHOD
Using a food processor, process the coconut for about 15 minutes (or, if you have a high-powered blender, about 2 minutes), until a runny butter forms. Scrape the sides of the bowl as necessary. Store in a jar either at room temperature or in the fridge, depending on the season and climate. Use as a soft spreadable paste on toast, sprinkled with salt—if you store the coconut butter in the fridge, you'll need to "cut out" a chunk and soften it at room temperature before using. Alternatively, melt and pour on a pancake with berries that you've simply stewed in their own juices.

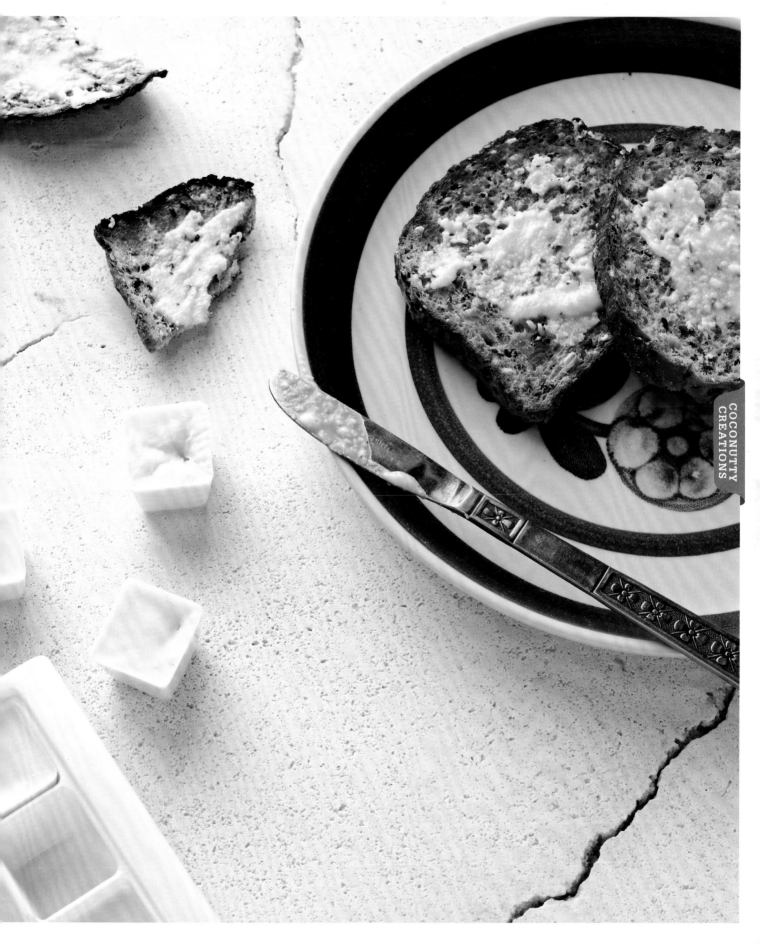

COCONUT CHOCOLATE BUTTER

You might want to make this in bulk and store it in ice-cube trays so you can pull out one or two for toast, pancakes or a smoothie, or for a little ganachey treat with your tea in the afternoon.

INGREDIENTS

3 tablespoons coconut oil, softened, at room temperature (or in the microwave for a few seconds)

1½ teaspoons raw cacao powder

2 tablespoons hazelnut meal (optional)

❄ **BATCH & FREEZE** | **SERVES** 2

METHOD

Using a teaspoon, mix all the ingredients in a small cup until blended (the cacao powder requires a bit of "smashing" to ensure all the lumps disappear). Refrigerate or freeze until firm.

"CARAMELIZED" COCONUT CHIPS

INGREDIENTS

1 cup unsweetened coconut flakes (the big chunky ones)

¼ teaspoon salt

pinch of ground cinnamon

MAKES 1 BIG BOWL

METHOD

Toast the flakes in a non-stick frying pan over medium–high heat for 2–3 minutes, until they are a nice toasty color. Stir frequently so they don't burn. Transfer to a bowl and toss with the salt and cinnamon. Allow to cool, then store in an airtight container.

CHOCOLATE COCONUT NUT BALLS

These balls are foolproof. A tip, though: the more you mix the nuts
and oil/butter, the better the balls will "hold."

COCONUTTY CREATIONS

INGREDIENTS

2½ cups nuts (almonds or brazil nuts are best),
preferably sprouted (see page 59)

½ cup almond butter

½ cup raw cacao powder (or to taste)

2 large handfuls of unsweetened shredded coconut

7–8 tablespoons salted butter, softened

4–5 heaped tablespoons coconut oil, softened, at room
temperature (or in the microwave for a few seconds)

vanilla powder or licorice root tea or granulated
stevia or ground cinnamon, to taste (choose the
flavor you prefer)

FILLERS (OPTIONAL)

almond meal, hempseed meal or other nut meal,
chia seeds, protein powder, maca powder,
acai powder

MAKES ABOUT 24

METHOD

Line a baking pan with baking paper. Roughly
chop the nuts in a food processor. Blend all the
ingredients in a bowl, using a metal spoon to
"smash" the coconut oil and butter through the dry
stuff. Don't be precise—throw in what feels right.
Add any fillers you have on hand or have a soft spot
for. The mixture will become quite wet because the
coconut oil will turn liquid. Add one or more of the
dry filler ingredients to adjust the consistency (chia
seeds do this super well) if you need or want to, and
if you happen to have them in the fridge. Grab small
handfuls, roll into balls and place on the pan. Stick
in the fridge for 1 hour to set before eating. The
balls will keep for several weeks in the fridge or
freezer.

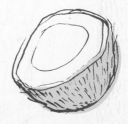

MY RASPBERRY RIPPLE

This would have to be one of the most popular recipes I've created. It's appeared on TV several times and has made cameos all over social media.

INGREDIENTS

⅓ cup frozen raspberries

⅓ cup unsweetened shredded coconut (or coconut flakes for a chunkier version)

⅓ cup coconut oil

5 tablespoons salted butter

2 tablespoons raw cacao powder or cocoa

2–3 tablespoons brown rice syrup

SERVES 6–8

METHOD

Line a dinner plate or baking pan with baking paper (a dinner plate is ideal as the slight indent creates a good shape). Scatter the berries and coconut on the plate or baking pan. Melt the oil and butter in a saucepan or in the microwave (the oil takes longer to melt, so add the butter a little after), then stir in the cacao powder and syrup. Pour over the berries and pop into the freezer for 30 minutes, until firm. To serve, either break into shards or cut into wedges.

NOTE
Be sure to use salted butter in this recipe—it gives a lovely kick.

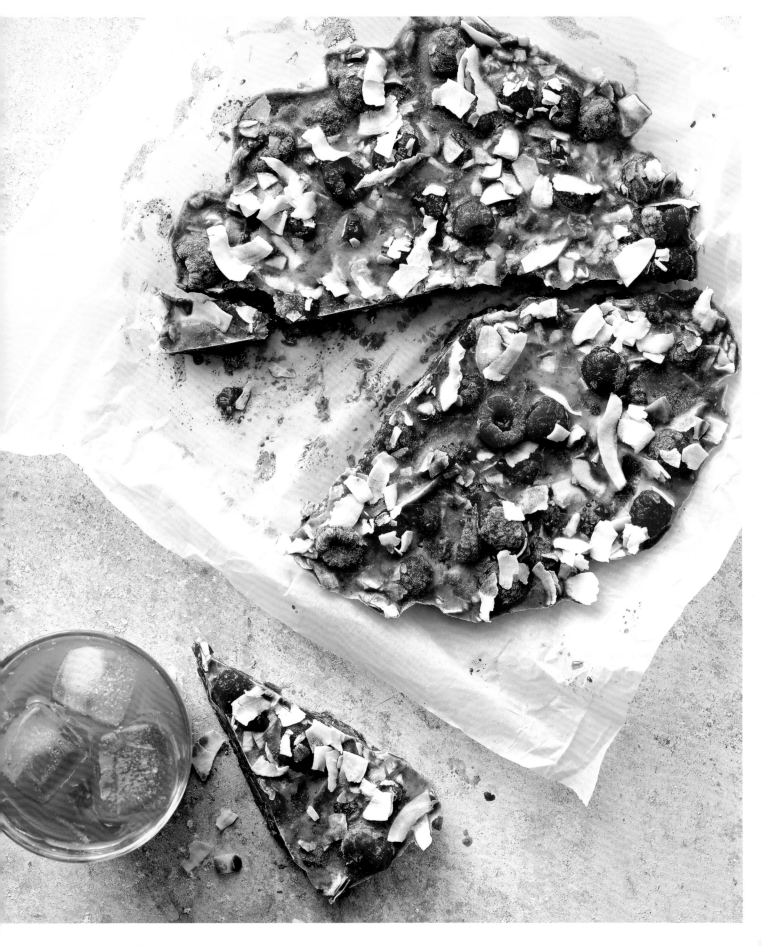

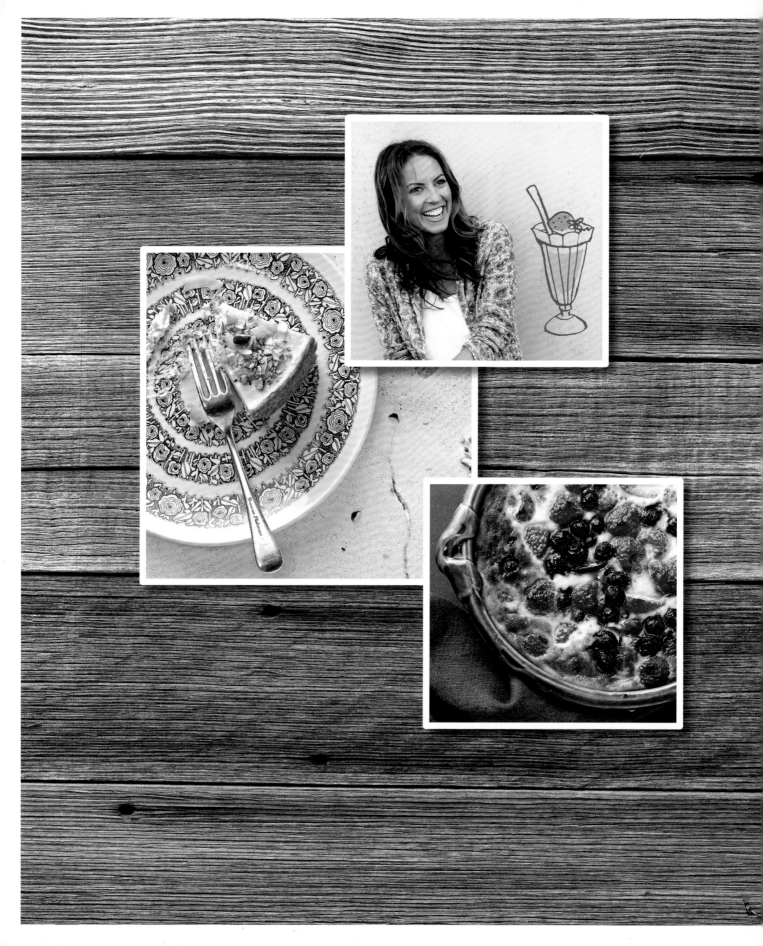

DESSERTS

⇨ **SOME PRETTY DESSERTS AND BAKED GOODNESS** ⇦

I've made all the recipes in this section for various special occasions, and they have never failed to convert a sugar addict or two. However, a little word before we start. Most of these contain sweeteners: fruit, brown rice syrup, dextrose or stevia. They're great as true treats—that is, occasional indulgences, so proceed with a little caution.

TIPS FOR: SAFE SWEETENERS

Now might be a good time to re-familiarize yourself with the various safe sugar alternatives and how much to use. They differ a lot. (See page 43 for details.)

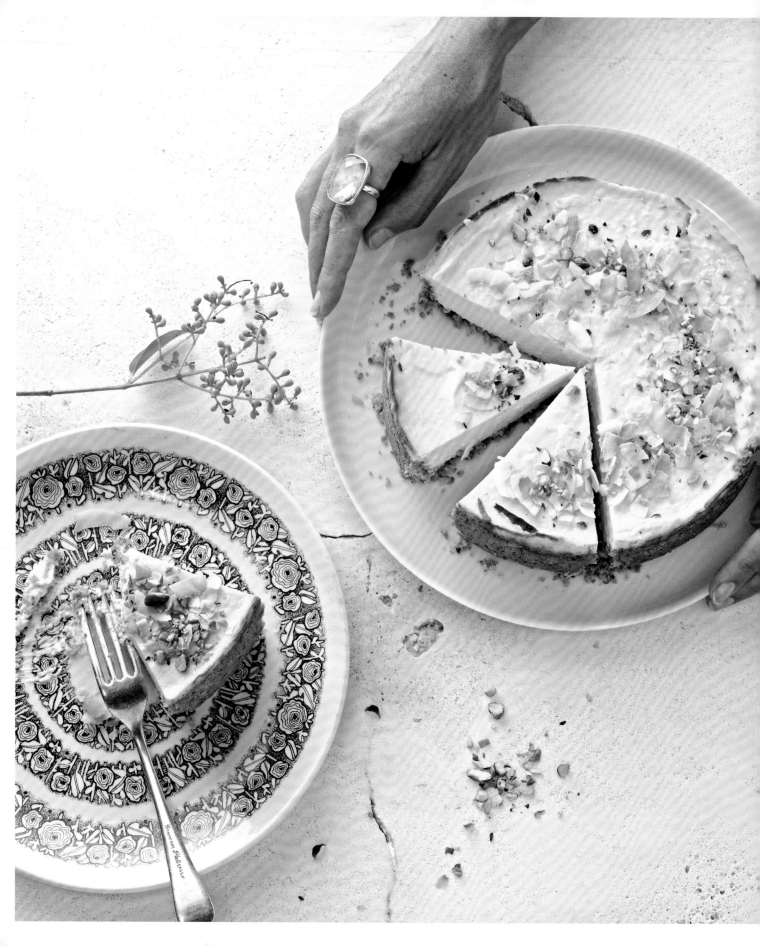

CRUNCHY-NUT CHEESECAKE

I made this cake one hot afternoon with my friend Claire. We just added bits of this and that until we got the right consistency. We dropped the base at one point (and mooshed it back together) and didn't have a temperature gauge on the oven, and still it worked out a treat. Proof that you can't screw it up! Be sure to allow the cheesecake to cool for several hours before serving; otherwise it can taste too eggy.

INGREDIENTS

CRUST
1 cup shelled pistachios or hazelnuts, sprouted, if possible
1 cup unsweetened shredded or desiccated coconut
1 cup almond meal, hempseed meal or other nut meal
8 tablespoons unsalted butter, softened

24 ounces homemade Cream Cheese (see page 64), at room temperature
2 tablespoons yogurt or sour cream
3 tablespoons coconut cream (see Note, page 167)
½ cup brown rice syrup (or to taste)
1 egg
dash of vanilla powder
small handful of pistachios and toasted unsweetened coconut flakes, to serve (optional)

SERVES 6–8

METHOD

Preheat the oven to 325°F and line the sides and bottom of a 9 in. springform pan with baking paper. To make the cheesecake crust, grind the nuts in a food processer until semi-fine. Add the coconut, almond meal and butter and rub with your fingers to make a dough. The more you rub, the more you'll release the oils in the nuts and achieve the right consistency. Add more butter if required. Press into the pan, covering the bottom and sides to an even thickness (about ¼ in.). Bake for 5–8 minutes, until starting to turn golden. Remove and allow to cool completely.

Combine the cream cheese, yogurt, coconut cream, syrup, egg and vanilla powder in a large bowl. Don't overmix, and try to keep the aeration to a minimum while stirring (too much air will make the filling puff up and then collapse during cooking). Spoon into the cold crust and return to the oven for 20–30 minutes or until the mixture pulls away from the crust a little and the center is custard-like (don't overcook). Place in the fridge for at least 2 hours to firm before serving. Sprinkle with pistachios and coconut flakes.

PUMPKIN PIE WITH CREAM

Don't be impatient when making this one. It's much better when it's cooked properly (it should look like a baked custard when you remove it from the oven). Also, be sure to leave it to cool for a good few hours (to allow it to set right). In fact, it's actually nicer the next day when it has set fully. It also works well frozen and thawed just a little.

INGREDIENTS

CRUST

4 tablespoons butter, melted

2 cups almond or hazelnut meal (or a combination of both, or use hempseed meal or other nut meal)

1 teaspoon salt

3 eggs

½ cup brown rice syrup

1½ cups canned unsweetened pumpkin purée or Squash Purée (see page 58)

¾ cup cream, plus extra to serve

1 tablespoon grated fresh ginger

1 teaspoon ground cinnamon

¼ teaspoon ground nutmeg

¼ teaspoon ground cloves

1 teaspoon salt

1–2 tablespoons arrowroot

grated zest of 1 lemon

SERVES 6–8

METHOD

Preheat the oven to 350°F. To make the crust, combine the melted butter, nut meal and salt in a 9 in. pie dish and mix well. (I find the crust "holds" better the more you work it, as this releases the oils in the nut meal.) Press the mixture into the bottom and up the sides of the dish to make a pie crust. If there isn't quite enough mixture, throw in a bit more of both butter and meal. Cook in the oven for 5–8 minutes, until it just starts to turn golden. Remove from the oven and let cool fully (refrigerate or freeze it if you are short of time).

Cream the eggs and syrup, then blend in the rest of the ingredients until the mixture is the consistency of thin custard. If it's a bit too runny, add extra arrowroot. Gently pour the filling into the cold crust and bake for 45–55 minutes or until the center of the pie is set (when it starts to pull away from the crust a little). Remove from the oven and allow to cool completely before putting in the fridge. Serve with cream (whipped, if desired).

⇨ *See variations on page 194.*

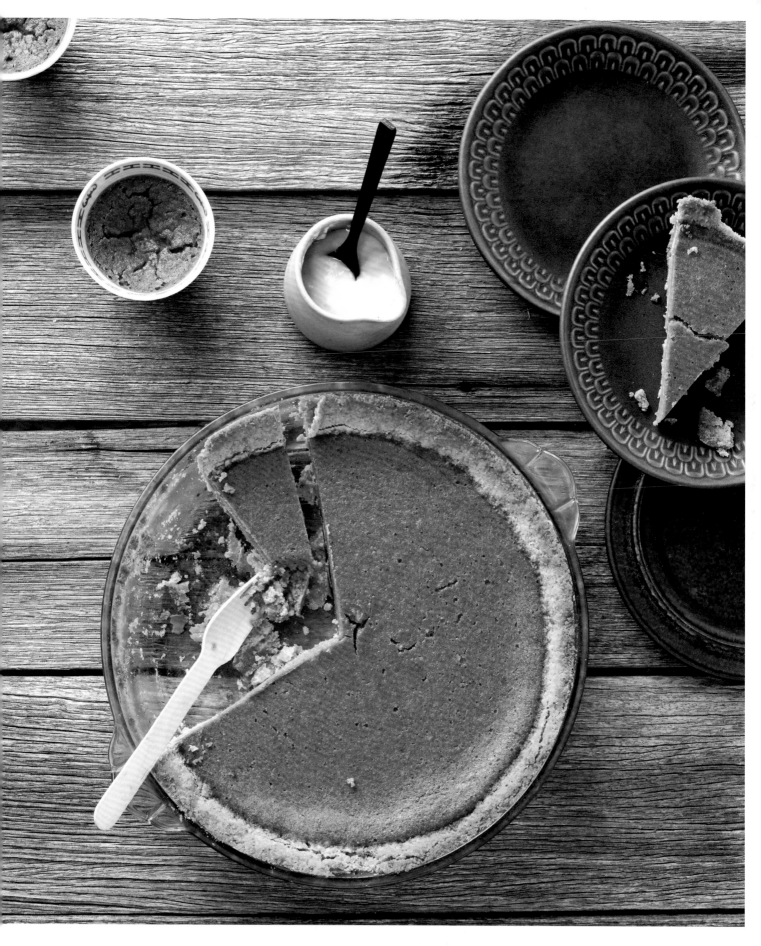

DAIRY-FREE PUMPKIN PIE WITH COCONUT

Make as for Pumpkin Pie with Cream (see page 192) but:

- use coconut oil instead of butter in the crust
- use less brown rice syrup (about 3 tablespoons)
- use coconut cream (see Note, page 167) instead of cream.

FIVE-SPICE PUMPKIN PIE

One clever thing: instead of the spices, you can use 1½ tablespoons of a five-spice mix that includes fennel and mandarin peel. I usually add an extra dose of ground cinnamon, too.

PUMPKIN PIE PUDDINGS WITH NUT CRUNCH

These are great for after-school snacks for the kids. Make up the filling as for Pumpkin Pie with Cream (see page 192). Pour into small ovenproof cups or ramekins and bake for 35–40 minutes, or until the centers of the puddings are set. Make a quarter of the amount of the crust mixture, spread on a baking pan and bake at the same time as the filling for 10 minutes, until golden. Sprinkle the crust on top of the puddings to serve. Cover any puddings you can't eat right away with plastic wrap and freeze.

MAKES 8–12 MINI PUDDINGS

NOTE

Instead of the nut crunch, you may wish to simply serve it with a spoonful of yogurt on top.

PEACHES WITH MELTED BŪCHERON

I first met celebrity chef Curtis Stone 15 years ago when he was surfing and eating his way around the globe. He's kindly shared this clever dessert that pairs cheese and relatively low-fructose fruit in full toasted glory!

INGREDIENTS

2 large ripe peaches, halved and pitted
four ½-inch-thick slices Būcheron cheese

SERVES 4

NOTE

Būcheron is a French goat cheese with an edible rind and the perfect diameter to cover a peach half. If you can't find it, use any soft goat cheese (with a diameter to cover the peach).

METHOD

Place the oven rack about 6 inches from the heat source and preheat the broiler. Line a heavy, rimmed baking sheet with aluminum foil.

Arrange the peach halves cut side up on the sheet and lay 1 slice of cheese over each peach half. Broil the peaches, watching closely, for about 45 seconds, or until the cheese melts and begins to brown. Serve immediately.

BLUEBERRY QUINOA CRUMBLE

INGREDIENTS

1 cup nuts and seeds (pecans, almonds, pumpkin seeds, sunflower kernels, sesame seeds—any combination will work)
1 cup cooked quinoa (see page 61)
¼ cup unsweetened shredded coconut
pinch salt
⅓ cup brown rice syrup
3 tablespoons butter or coconut oil, melted
3–4 cups fresh or frozen blueberries
½ teaspoon vanilla powder (optional)
yogurt, to serve

SERVES 6–8

METHOD

Preheat the oven to 350°F. Using a food processer, roughly chop the nuts and seeds (they should still be a little chunky). Add the quinoa, coconut and salt and pulse a few times to combine. Combine the syrup and butter in a large bowl, then add the quinoa mixture and stir. Arrange the berries in a baking dish, sprinkle with vanilla powder and scatter the quinoa mixture over. Bake for 20 minutes, until golden. Serve warm with yogurt.

LAVENDER ICE CREAM AND BLUEBERRY SUNDAE

People—including me—travel far to sample Sarma Melngailis's ice cream.
It's legendary stuff and I'm honored that she's agreed to share this very special
recipe with me, allowing me to give it a little I Quit Sugar makeover. Sarma suggests
sourcing your lavender at greenmarkets. If you can't find it, use chamomile (and
team it with a blackberry version of the sauce) or mint (with strawberries). If you
don't have an ice-cream maker, pour the mixture into an ice cream container and
place it in the freezer. After 1 to 2 hours, mix with an immersion blender,
then return it to the freezer for another hour. Blend again, then store in the freezer
until you're ready to serve.

INGREDIENTS

2 cups raw cashews, soaked 4 hours or more
2 cups coconut meat
1 cup filtered water
¾ cup brown rice syrup
½ cup coconut butter (storebought, or make your own, see page 182)
2 tablespoons edible organic lavender flowers
2 teaspoons vanilla extract (or 1½ teaspoons of vanilla powder)
½ teaspoon sea salt
1 cup Berry Grown-Up Sauce (see page 68; use only blueberries if possible)
½ cup Candied Pecans (see page 174)
Lemon basil leaves or sprigs of lavender for garnish

SERVES 4–6

METHOD

In a high-powered blender, blend the cashews, coconut meat, water, brown rice syrup, coconut butter, lavender, vanilla and sea salt until completely smooth. Chill thoroughly in the refrigerator and then process in an ice cream maker according to the manufacturer's instructions. Serve with the Berry Grown-Up Sauce and the pecans.

NOTE
Coconut meat is the white flesh scraped from the inside of a baby (also called "green") coconut, available at some health food shops and supermarkets. If you can't find these in your neighborhood, you can substitute 1 can of chilled coconut cream and either ½ cup of unsweetened coconut flakes or an additional 2 tablespoons of coconut butter.

AVOCADO AND CHOCOLATE MOUSSE

I like to experiment with this recipe—for example, you might like
it with less cacao powder. The chia seeds make it nice and thick and
have a texture like chocolate chips.

INGREDIENTS

2 ripe avocados

½ cup chilled coconut cream (see Note, page 167;
it needs to be firm)

¼–½ cup raw cacao powder

1 tablespoon chia seeds

1–2 teaspoons granulated stevia, or
2 teaspoons brown rice syrup

1 teaspoon vanilla extract or a sprinkle of vanilla powder

½ teaspoon ground cinnamon

pinch of sea salt

SERVES 4–6

METHOD

Whiz all the ingredients in a blender until smooth.
Scoop the mousse into small serving dishes, such
as antique teacups (I use little Chinese teacups),
and put in the fridge to chill for at least 2 hours.

CHOCOLATE BERRY MUD

This chocolaty dessert is gloriously simple and 100% nutritious, and it tastes as good as any sorbet I've eaten—perhaps a little creamier, even! You can use the quantities given here to make 4 smaller servings, if you prefer. Pour into little teacups and freeze, then you can pull 1 out, let it thaw for about an hour, and eat on a hot afternoon when you "need" chocolate.

INGREDIENTS

½ cup frozen berries
½ medium ripe avocado
1 cup baby spinach leaves
¼ cup raw cacao powder
½ teaspoon granulated stevia
pinch of vanilla powder
2 trays ice cubes

SERVES 2

METHOD

Blend all the ingredients using a blender, preferably a high-powered one. If you're using a regular blender or an immersion blender, add a little water. Pour into bowls and serve immediately.

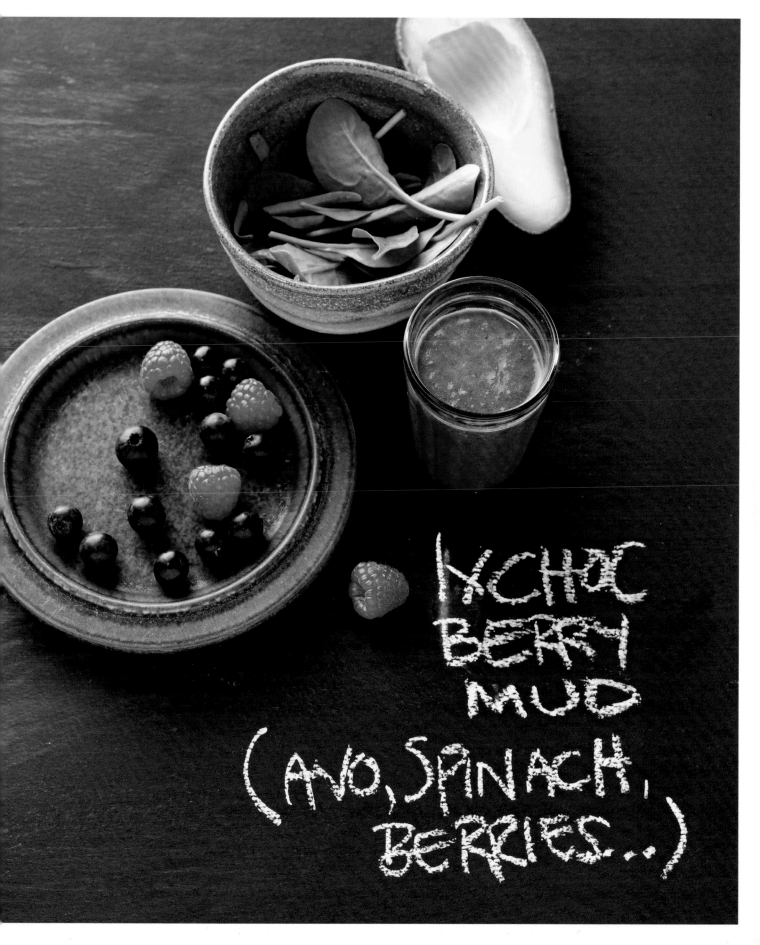

NCHOC
BERRY
MUD
(AVO, SPINACH,
BERRIES...)

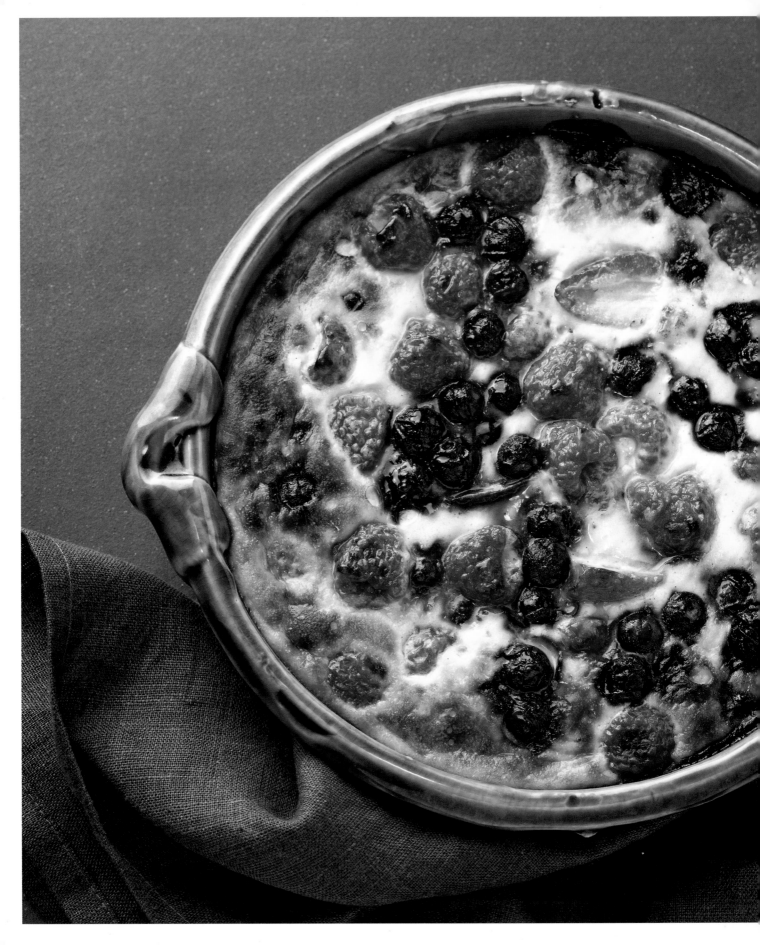

BERRIES WITH CARAMELIZED CREAM

Gwyneth Paltrow kindly shared this recipe with me. She says she invented it as a
fridge surprise when she didn't have time to make a cobbler, saying, "I just adjusted
the sweetener." It takes her 7 minutes to make, she reckons. Time yourself!

INGREDIENTS

2 pints blueberries, blackberries and/or raspberries
9 ounces mascarpone
2 tablespoons sour cream
2 tablespoons heavy cream
1 large egg, plus 1 egg white extra
3 tablespoons granulated stevia
seeds from 1 vanilla bean
pinch of salt

SERVES 4–6

METHOD

Put the oven rack in the middle or lower half of the
oven and preheat the broiler. Put the berries in a
pie dish or casserole dish. Whisk together the
remaining ingredients until completely smooth,
then pour over the berries. Put the dish under
the broiler and cook for 5–10 minutes, until the
topping is just browned and caramelized. Serve
immediately.

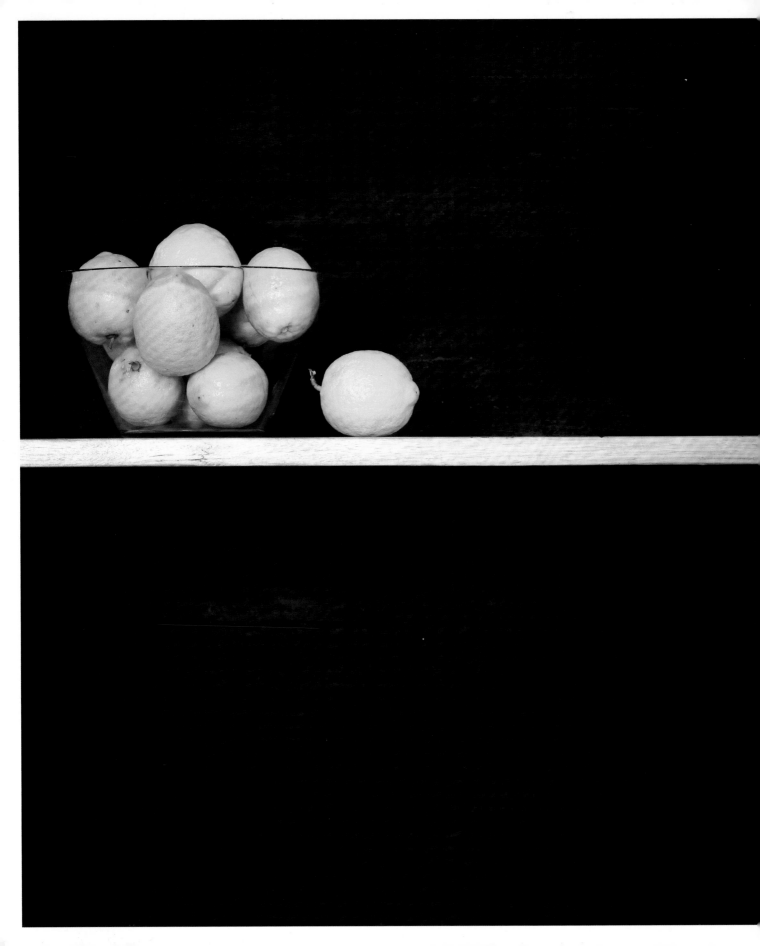

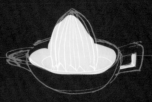

THE BITS AT THE BACK OF THE BOOK

THE SHOPPING LIST

This is not a comprehensive list of ingredients and it doesn't include fresh produce. It's the stuff that's best to have on hand when quitting sugar (for quick snacks and the like) and for cooking the bulk of the recipes.

PLEASE REMEMBER THIS!

I've streamlined things so there's no waste or superfluous, random ingredients you'll never use again!

IN YOUR PANTRY

- Chia seeds
- Canned tuna and other canned fish
- Ground cinnamon
- Sea salt
- Unsweetened oconut flakes
- Vanilla: I like to use the powder (organic), but extract form is okay.

IN YOUR FRIDGE

- Haloumi cheese (choose organic varieties where possible; store leftover chunks in a container filled with water)
- Other types of unprocessed cheese: I like to work with goat's cheese quite a bit—it goes well with nuts and cinnamon. But your choice.
- Nut butter: macadamia, almond, peanut (not the processed kind), cashew. Buy one at a time and work out which one you like best.
- Tahini
- Eggs. always free-range organic
- Yogurt: full-fat and unflavored. Try different types—Greek styles, sheep's milk, goat's milk.
- Avocados
- Sliced/shaved meat: chicken, turkey, ham
- Coconut water
- Coconut cream (see Note, page 167; yes, best stored in the fridge!)
- Organic butter (never margarine)

IN YOUR FREEZER

- Sprouted nuts (see page 59)
- Vegetables: broccoli, beets squash, onion (see page 59)
- Frozen berries

OILS

- Coconut
- Olive
- Nut oils: this is optional, but you might like to try some of the "sweeter" varieties, like macadamia oil (my favorite) for pouring over yogurt, cheese, vegetables.

CONDIMENTS

- Mustard: yellow, whole-grain, Dijon—your choice
- Mayonnaise: whole egg only
- Tamari
- Apple cider vinegar

SWEETENERS

- Brown rice syrup
- Stevia: I recommend finding a granulated version that can be used in a 1:1 manner.

TEAS

- Chai
- Dandelion or rooibos
- Herbal blends containing cinnamon, fennel, nutmeg, liquorice
- Green tea

BAKING BITS

- Coconut flour
- Raw cacao powder

RESOURCES

WHERE TO BUY HARD-TO-FIND INGREDIENTS

If you're having trouble sourcing some of the items in this book such as the supplement powders
on page 69, the alternate sweeteners, or even coconut oil or stevia,
these online stores should be able to help:

Amazon.com   **Nuts.com**

Bobsredmill.com (buckwheat groats)   **Swansonvitamins.com**

Globalsugarart.com (glucose syrup)   **The BakersKitchen.net (glucose syrup)**

iHerb.com   **Vitacost.com**

LiveSuperfoods.com   **VitaminShoppe.com**

Luckyvitamin.com

My NaturalMarket.com

A FEW SPECIAL FOLKS KINDLY KICKED IN A SUGAR-FREE RECIPE.

If you liked their creation, you should check out their respective books, blogs and bytes.

⇨ SARAH BRITTON

A Copenhagen-based holistic nutritionist and vegetarian chef—and an incredibly sweet and generous soul to boot—Sarah is the creative force behind award-winning blog My New Roots and is currently on assignment at Noma's test kitchen, the Nordic Food Lab. A certified nutritional practitioner, Sarah is also founder of New Roots Holistic Nutrition.

⇨ JOE CROSS

Joe is a New York–based media entrepreneur. I met Joe several years ago and have stayed in contact since, getting updates on his Reboot Media project—a health and lifestyle brand that makes juices (available in supermarkets) and cookbooks and educates on getting well. (Joe was fat, tired and seriously sick when we met and he healed himself through his eating alone!) Make sure you look out for his film *Fat, Sick and Nearly Dead*. The guy's an inspiration!

⇨ SALLY FALLON

Sally is a Washington-based journalist, chef and nutrition researcher. She's also founder of the Weston A. Price Foundation for Wise Traditions in Foods, which educates on eating whole foods with plenty of good fats and protein. Her book *Nourishing Traditions: The Cookbook That Challenges Politically Correct Nutrition and the Diet Dictocrats* not only has the best subtitle ever, it's my most cherished cookbook.

⇨ ARAN GOYOAGA

Aran is a a Basque food stylist now based in the U.S., is the beautiful writer and chef behind the blog *Cannelle et Vanille*. We met online and connected via our shared issues with thyroid disease. We've never met but we write to each other on Twitter and email. A modern pen pal kind of thing. Her cookbook *Small Plates and Sweet Treats* is full of elegant, creative and nutritious food, which is gluten free and easily adapted to be sugar free, too.

ANGELA LIDDON

Angela is the Canada-based creator of Oh She Glows, an incredibly popular healthy vegan recipe website. Her work has been featured in O, *Fitness, Self, Veg News, Glamour, Glow* and *Best Health*. *Chatelaine Magazine* named her one of Canada's Women of the Year 2011. She's currently working on her first vegan cookbook for release in 2014.

DR. ROBERT LUSTIG

Dr. Robert Lustig is a San Francisco–based pediatric endocrinologist and the man behind the consciousness-shifting YouTube hit *Sugar: The bitter truth*. His latest book Fat Chance: The Bitter Truth About Sugar turns our understanding of obesity on its head and points the finger squarely at . . . sugar.

SARMA MELNGAILIS

Sarma is the owner and co-founder of the Pure Food and Wine raw food restaurant in New York City, and the founder and CEO of One Lucky Duck. A passionate vegan, she's also incredibly open and, um, raw, about her wellness approach. I love this. She is honest about the fact that she is still learning and still struggling . . . but makes the best choices she can, when she can. She's published two very popular popular books, *Raw Food Real World* and *Living Raw Food*.

GWYNETH PALTROW

Gwyneth needs little introduction. But perhaps you haven't checked out her cookbook *Notes from My Kitchen Table* yet? With a breezy and generous spirit, similar to the vibe of her site Goop, she shares 150 of her favorite recipes, how she involves her kids in cooking and how she balances healthy food with homemade treats.

MARK SISSON

Mark is a California-based blogger and health guru. His site Mark's Daily Apple is the go-to joint for Paleo living. Mark's *Primal Blueprint Cookbook* is available through his website.

CURTIS STONE

Curtis is a chef, author and TV personality who hosts *Top Chef Masters*. His philosophy is to cook as Mother Nature intended—buy local, seasonal and organic ingredients, keep recipes simple and allow the food to speak for itself. His latest cookbook *What's For Dinner?* is super clever and 100% accessible, geared at families and everyone wanting to minimize waste.

PAGE REFERENCES IN *ITALICS* INDICATE PHOTOGRAPHS.

ACKNOWLEDGMENTS

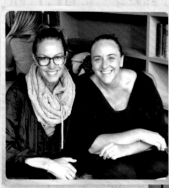

← Jo ... on the right!

Marija and I toasting →
the end of another great
photo shoot—in Copenhagen!

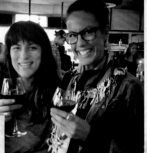

↑
Faustina and Lee→

I'm grateful to the readers on my blog who encouraged my sugar-free experimenting and steered me to turning it into a book.

I'd also like to thank **Jo Foster** for being there, just to my right, ready to go, always.

And **Marija Ivkovic** for her supreme picture work and for flying to the other side of the planet to support me. Quite literally.

Love, also, to **Faustina, Lee, Trisha,** and **Lisa Valuyskaya** for their fervor and skill.

And to the Pan Macmillan team in Australia and the warm, encouraging and embracing team at Clarkson Potter in the U.S. Thank you for "seeing my message."

Oh (is the band starting up yet?), thank you to **my Mum**.

For showing me how to love food.
xx

ABOUT THE AUTHOR

Sarah Wilson is an Australian media personality, journalist, health coach and blogger. She's the former editor of *Cosmopolitan* magazine and was the host of the first series of *MasterChef Australia*, the highest-rating show in Australian TV history, as well as the health makeover series *Eat Yourself Sexy*. She kicked off her career as a restaurant reviewer for NewsCorp, then moved into political and social commentary, appearing regularly on Australian screens as a host on a number of Australian morning shows and a regular panelist on current affairs programs.

She's also been a regular magazine and newspaper columnist for over a decade, a gig that's seen her

MEDITATE WITH THE DALAI LAMA, TAP DANCE OUT OF A PLANE WITH SIR RICHARD BRANSON AND DISCUSS DATING TIPS WITH THE PRIME MINISTER OF AUSTRALIA.

Sarah likes biking, hiking and wearing the same pair of green shorts (for eight years; she's not quite sure why). She's come full circle now, focusing again on food with her *I Quit Sugar* book and website iquitsugar.com.

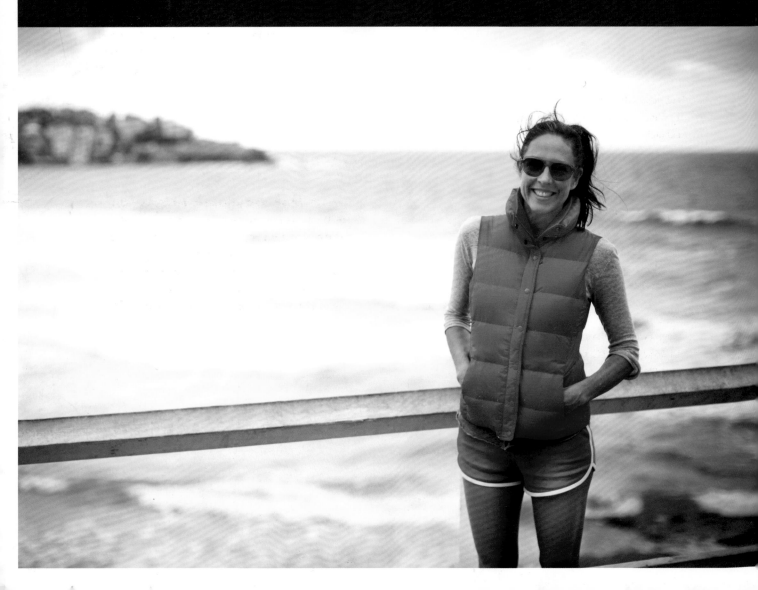